Please return

Les Howard

248 623 1009

howaussie @ comcast.net

Crossing Divides

Crossing Divides

*A Couple's Story of Cancer,
Hope, and Hiking
Montana's
Continental Divide*

SCOTT BISCHKE
Foreword by Katie Gibson

American Cancer Society
Health Content Products
1599 Clifton Road NE
Atlanta, Georgia 30329, USA

Cover photo digital illustration by Dana Wagner.
Designed by Barbara Werden Design, Lubbock, Texas.

Chapter 2 quote from Walkin' Jim Stoltz's "All Along the Great Divide":
© 1984 Walkin' Jim Stoltz, Walkin' Jim Music/BMI

Chapter 4, Dr. George Sheehan's quote: from one of his *Runner's World* essays:
© The George Sheehan Trust

Chapter 11 quote from TR Ritchie's "Changing of the Guard": © 1990 Whitebark Music/BMI

Epilogue quote from Christine Lavin's "Bumblebees":
Bumblebees Words and Music by Christine Lavin
Copyright © 1992 CL2 Music (ASCAP), DreamWorks Songs (ASCAP) and Rounder Music (ASCAP) Worldwide Rights for CL2 Music and DreamWorks Songs Administered by Cherry Lane Music Publishing Company, Inc. International Copyright Secured
ALL RIGHTS RESERVED

In a few minor instances, names have been changed so that Katie and Scott could share candid thoughts from people they encountered along their health and/or hiking journeys.

5 4 3 2 1 02 03 04 05 06

Library of Congress Cataloging-in-Publication Data
Bischke, Scott, 1959-
Crossing divides : a couple's story of cancer, hope, and hiking Montana's continental divide / by Scott Bischke; foreword by Katie Gibson.
p. cm.
ISBN 0-944235-39-5
1. Gibson, Katie, 1962—-Health. 2. Bischke, Scott, 1959- 3. Cervix uteri—Patients—United States—Biography. 4. Hiking—Montana. 5. Hiking—Continental Divide National Scenic Trail. 6. Continental Divide National Scenic Trail. I. Title.
RC280.U8 B55 2002
362.1'9699466—dc21

2001006182

Printed in the United States of America

MANAGING EDITOR
Katherine Bruss, Psy.D.

EDITOR
Amy Sproull Brittain

EDITORIAL REVIEW
Terri Ades, R.N., M.S., A.O.C.N.
Rick Alteri, M.D.

EDITORIAL DIRECTOR
Chuck Westbrook

PUBLISHING DIRECTOR
Diane Scott-Lichter

BOOK PUBLISHING MANAGER
Candace Magee

CONTENTS

MAPS

FOREWORD

◪

IT'S BEEN A MONTH since my husband Scott and I got home from another summer of hiking—this time down the Continental Divide Trail (CDT) of Colorado. We completed the Wyoming CDT last year, and now we only have to walk one more state—New Mexico—to complete the 3,100-mile trail. During this summer's hike we had some amazing animal encounters, including seeing a herd of 150 elk running over the grassy divide and spotting bears, coyotes, a few moose, and a badger. Our hike through Colorado often followed right along the Divide ridge and took us over peaks of 13,000 and 14,000 feet.

After cancer and recurrent cancer, I feel lucky just to be alive, much less able to hike down this wonderful trail through the Rockies. At first it was hard to accept that cancer had been thrust into my life. Once, after I was diagnosed, I walked out of a movie theater feeling happy, then suddenly remembered that I supposedly only had a short time to live. My heart sank to its lowest possible level and I felt a sense of hopelessness. There was no way to prepare for such a drastic change in my outlook on life. I wanted a reason to be happy, but the cancer acted like an anchor, weighing me down.

Some doctors suggested that I consider not having treatment because they believed my cancer could not be cured. Others advised that I pursue various treatments. There were both optimists and pessimists around me, and in the end *I* had to weigh all the research, opinions, and my own gut feelings in order to decide which direction I wanted to go in. That is one idea I hope you will take away from this book: You and only you are responsible for deciding your path.

Because several of the cancer books I read while exploring treatment options suggested doing visualization, I thought I would give it a try. One day I visualized myself getting well—I saw all of the cancer cells dying, my body's health taking over, and visualized myself completely healthy again. All of a sudden I felt a wave of freedom, as though I could actually do something about getting well. The something I could do was to believe in the possibility that *I could get well*. After that realization I felt so much happier. I decided that living with possibility was better than living without hope.

Scott and I received a lot of support from the people around us. The doctors and nurses who took care of me during cancer treatments acted in truly kind ways. Our friends spoke to us from their hearts, making us feel loved. Our family members visited regularly and checked on us to see if we were okay. All of these things helped us to be strong. Scott was in this with me from day one. He never spoke in a way that separated him from my medical problems. He always assumed that cancer was his problem to solve, too. I felt his incredible support and that he was part of the ups and downs with me. (Although I do admit feeling some jealousy when he got to go out for Mexican food at dinnertime and I had to stay in my hospital bed. I try not to hold it against him.)

In our lives before cancer, Scott and I loved doing almost anything outdoors. We felt enlivened and recharged when we came home from a hike or a canoe trip or a bike ride in a beautiful place. Memories of these kinds of places provided me with a mental refuge when I was working toward getting well. In times of pain I mentally escaped to my favorite places in the outdoors—hiking in the Rockies with the sun on my back, pedaling my bicycle on a dirt road through the New Zealand bush, or sea kayaking down an awesome river in Alaska seeing bear, salmon, and seals. If I could get back outside again, I thought, breathe fresh air, and feel the warmth of the sun, I would appreciate it even more than I ever had before.

People get their strength in many different ways. Sometimes remembering a great experience, thinking of a peaceful place, or dreaming of how you'd like things to be in the future can make you feel better. I hope that you will find your own dream to hold on to and that this dream will help you get through treatment and on to living.

It was a blessing that we were able to hike down the Continental Divide Trail of Montana after my cancer experience. The hiking parts of this story show the joy (and sometimes exhaustion) we felt as we made our way through Montana. In the first few days we were in awe of just being out there. After a couple of bear encounters we felt fear and questioned why we were there. Maybe it sounds crazy for us to have spent years getting me well from cancer, only to go out into grizzly bear country. But we wanted to be back in the wild country that I dreamed of when things were at their worst.

So many events and emotions are tied up together in my cancer experience over the last nine years. I want to share that experience in an effort to help others, especially those who might be dealing with cancer or supporting someone with cancer. You may feel hopelessness, fear, impatience, and anxiety over your treatment, as I did. Please know you're not alone. In the story that follows, Scott shares our emotions and dreams; perhaps you will relate to them. Scott tells our story carefully, at times humorously, reflecting as closely as possible what happened. He shares his thoughts and feelings through the story and weaves in mine. My hope is that reading about our experience will help you better deal with how cancer has affected your life.

When battling cancer, I wished for a simple set of rules to live by, but there were none. I had to find my own path, and I continue to do so today. I wish I could hand you a recipe for getting well, but I can't. What I can do is, with Scott, share our story in hopes that you will find similarities to your own situation and somehow gain hope and inspiration. My biggest hope is for you to be empowered to find out the information you need, to make decisions as best you can, and to not be afraid.

I realized during my cancer experience that each of us has a hundred times more strength than we realize. This strength helps us get through seemingly impossible moments. May you find this strength and use it to guide you along your path to well-being.

Katie Gibson

PREFACE

◪

The point was the most dangerous place. . . . It was also a great confluence of life, and this combination of peril and substance sent the spirit spinning off into various ethereal regions, in which a man might be tempted to commit philosophy.

TIM CAHILL
Pecked to Death by Ducks

THIS BOOK has a simple purpose: We hope our story can help others who are newly diagnosed with cancer or some other debilitating disease, and those who support them. We hope our story will offer others hope.

When we learned Kate had cancer, we felt nothing but despair. We agonized. We cried. We got mad. Then, as the hard edge of our initial emotions softened, we began to study and question and search for answers, both in the medical world and in our own souls.

And we read. We read a lot. Medical journals bolstered our knowledge of the cancer and, as importantly, what medical science did and did not know about how to treat the disease. Less technical books helped too, we found, especially those about real people who had faced cancer or other afflictions.

Kate is a private person. She is not prone to participating in support groups. While many gain strength from such groups, neither Kate nor I felt drawn to them. But books offered us another way to learn about other people's struggles and successes. Books allowed us to learn from others without the emotional ties of new relationships that might absorb much of Kate's precious energy. Perhaps this approach was selfish, but for us it was very, very necessary. We had quickly discovered that getting well from cancer is not a part-time occupation. Anything that shifted our focus from the primary goal of getting well had no place in our plan to survive cancer. Surviving cancer demanded—and continues to demand— our full presence.

Because of Kate's bent toward privacy, the idea of sharing our own experience took a great deal of thought, a great deal of soul searching. At the suggestion of a friend we have written journals through much of our healing time. As Kate's health has improved over the years, the entries into those journals have come further and further apart. The pain is still close, however, and as we began this book, I did not know if we would be able to share our innermost thoughts, fears, and memories, or if—in the end—the process would simply be too painful. That pain proved tangible; I know I cried many times when I read back through our journals.

I also know that this process was harder on Kate than on me. I am the writer in the family, so we knew that if we were to convey our story it would be up to me. But while Kate has prodded and pulled the pages during the preparation of this manuscript, added her memories, and reshaped mine, reliving the past nine years has been especially tough on her. Living with cancer is immediate and forward, requiring a focus on today and tomorrow. The act of pulling our old memories back to the surface hurts.

It is *our* story because we both accept the changes cancer caused in our lives and we both accept the challenge to do anything and everything necessary to get well from cancer. But physically it was Kate's cancer. I can share the fears, but I cannot and would not pretend that I have suffered the way Kate has. I cannot take away the anguish of the treatments she suffered through. I cannot take away her swelling legs or her struggles with a malfunctioning bladder and bowel.

We have been blessed to have Kate cancer-free for over six years. During those years we have worked hard to regain a sense of freedom and to reclaim a world of limitless possibilities. So much of our joy has always come from the natural world; the howl of the wolf, the feel of cold wind off an icy stream, the deep blue of twilight all resonate in us. During one of our worst moments with cancer, a moment when life seemed to be ebbing away, Kate remarked sadly, "It upsets me to think that I might not be able to go back to some of the awesome places we've been, that we might not be able to hike or canoe or explore together anymore."

And so we have incorporated our love of the outdoors into our healing plan. We have sea kayaked and canoed and bicycled and backpacked in some "awesome" places, both near home and far away.

On a cellular basis, the cancer is gone. But recovering from cancer entails so much more: a loss of innocence, a change of focus, a need to rebuild. Life changes after cancer, and many of those changes are good. We have grown deeper friendships. We have taken control of and responsibility for our lives. We have redoubled our commitment to the purity of physical exercise. We have embraced simplicity. We have learned that we hold a special love for a special place—Montana. And we have learned to value our time for what it is: a precious, limited commodity.

Around Christmas 1997, nearly three years after Kate's final cancer treatment, we threw all of these things into a blender. The concoction that resulted was a plan for a north-to-south walk across the state of Montana along the Continental Divide Trail. We didn't know if Kate's health was sufficient for her to carry a pack over 900 miles that following summer. We did know that we wanted to accept the lives we now had, and that we wanted to live our lives without fearing that even in its absence, cancer might control us.

Five hundred miles into our journey across Montana the following summer, shortly after walking out of the Anaconda–Pintler Wilderness, Kate decided that if our story could help someone else, the resulting loss of privacy would not matter. And so I would like to tell you about our hike across Montana, and our ongoing journey to well-being.

Scott Bischke

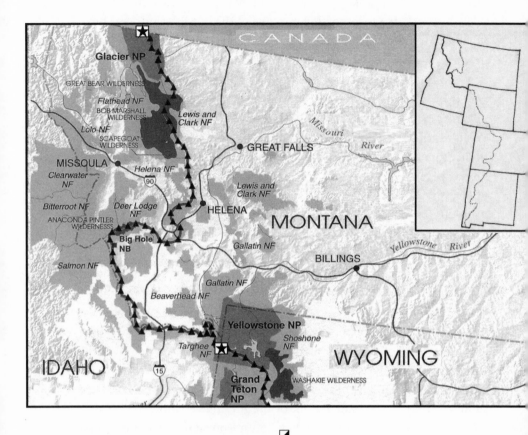

Overview of the Continental Divide as it crosses Montana. The star at the top of the map indicates the northernmost point of the Continental Divide Trail and the start of our hike. The star at the Yellowstone National Park boundary shows where our hike ended. The inset shows the entire 3,100 miles of the Continental Divide Trail as it traverses the United States.

Map courtesy of Continental Divide Trail Alliance, www.cdtrail.org

Crossing Divides

ONE

Enter the Bear

*One of his favorite remarks was
"if you know what a bear is going to do next,
you know more than the bear does."*

FRANK DUFRESNE
No Room for Bears

U NLIKE MOST PEOPLE, Kate and I can tell you the exact day we entered "middle age," a day in December of 1992. Middle age, to me, has nothing to do with chronological age. Instead middle age describes the transition from a world of limitless opportunity to one suddenly fringed with boundaries. I left my youth behind just moments after Kate left hers, when I picked up the phone at work and she blurted out, "The doctor just called and said I have cancer."

Kate's voice at once sounded of fear, disbelief, and confusion. I reacted as you might expect, saying, "What? Cancer? You can't possibly have cancer! You're 30 years old. What did he say? Something must be wrong."

Unfortunately, something *was* wrong. During a normal checkup, Kate's gynecologist had discovered a three-centimeter mass on her cervical wall. A biopsy, just completed, had shown the mass to be malignant. Since Kate and I worked at the same company, we quickly met up and went home. The doctor agreed to see us in an hour to explain the results of the biopsy.

I recall little about that meeting when we first faced cancer besides

1

being filled with disbelief. Two months earlier we had run the Victoria Marathon. Kate had always been a vigorous outdoorswoman, a near vegetarian, a health nut to the nth degree. Cancer? Kate? Moose poop!

Three things about that meeting I do recall, vividly. The first we did not understand, "papillary adenocarcinoma." The second rang cold and clear: "This could be very serious," the doctor said. *"This could kill you."* The third was Kate and me departing the hospital feeling as though we'd just been kicked in the chest.

◪

Skip forward one month into our hike across Montana, to July 1998.

Kneeling in the tent I heard Kate's voice in the distance yelling, "Go away!" Must be a chipmunk, I thought; they always bedevil her. Our tent sat on a bench high above the West Fork of the Sun River, in the Bob Marshall Wilderness. While I was changing clothes after fishing, Kate had gone to our cook area to start dinner.

"Go away!" I heard again. This time it sounded more urgent. *"Get out of here!"*

I grabbed my pepper spray, somewhat melodramatically I recall thinking, and emerged from the tent. At that same moment Kate shouted, "Scott, there's a *bear* over here!" From a hundred yards away I could see the bear sitting on its haunches, just ten steps from Kate, facing her. Though a fire smoked, our food still hung in the tree above and to the left of Kate. The bear looked like the same bear we'd seen on the trail hours earlier, the reason we'd turned around and quit early for the day.

"What do you want me to do?" I yelled. Kate paused in amazement, clearly contemplating how she had ended up marrying such an unchivalrous dolt. For its part, the ponderous beast looked my way and then stood on its hind legs, trying to scent or see this new intrusion. Kate and the bear now stood eye to eye, the bear between her and me. From my vantage point, it looked like two steps forward and they could easily do a do-si-do.

"Don't worry," Kate yelled over the bear's shoulder. Her voice sounded surprisingly calm. "It's a black bear, not a grizzly."

"Are you sure?" I yelled back, dismally failing to reclaim any valor.

Black bears, we both knew, tend to be less dangerous than grizzlies. Another thing we both knew—something that was painfully apparent— was that this bear was honey blonde, a common color for grizzlies.

"I'm sure." Her tone had turned flat and somewhat defiant. For its part the bear continued to stand on its hind legs, face quizzical, glancing between Kate and me as if watching a tennis match.

"Don't come up the trail," Kate shouted finally. For a moment I thought she was insinuating that she would be better off battling the beast by herself, but then she added, "That would push him toward me. Come up the gully."

I grabbed some rocks and jogged down into the gully. Our shouted conversation and my disappearance apparently convinced the bear to change plans. It dropped uncertainly back on all fours. After looking longingly at the empty pot near the fire, the bear waddled off. "He's leaving," Kate yelled, and then a moment later as I emerged from the gully, she called out, "No, no, he's still here."

By the time I reached Kate, the blonde bear stood 20 yards away in sparse forest. We both hollered at him and Kate banged our pot with a tree branch. The bear watched us, unimpressed. Together Kate and I threw rocks, and the bear moved two more steps up onto the hillside. And then, glancing back and throwing us a yawn, the bear lay down!

Kate and I exchanged stupefied looks. "Okay, great, now what are we supposed to do?"

We tossed more rocks and finally I nailed the bear hard on the rear end. That brought him to his feet, now facing us, ears laid back, shoulders low, snarling.

"That can't be a good thing," Kate whispered, wide-eyed.

"Maybe we ought to back out of here," I proposed. But before we could move, the bear, snarling once more, pointed itself up the hill and moved stiffly away.

As the bear disappeared and reappeared among the trees, I said, "That could be a griz."

"It's a black bear!" Kate snapped back. "It stood right in front of me. It doesn't have a shoulder hump. Besides, look how small it is."

"Small?" The bear I saw looked big enough to play defensive end for Chicago.

*   *   *

Talking with a backcountry ranger the next morning, Kate, her face animated and unafraid, described the encounter: "I looked up from the fire to see the bear, sneaking up on its belly just like a dog would. It was sniffing, so I figured it wanted food. The bear seemed kind of scared, so at first I just sat there trying to decide what I should do. When it kept coming, I knew I had to grab my bear spray, stand up, and scare it away. . . ."

As Kate talked on, I realized her story was not unlike our encounter with cancer.

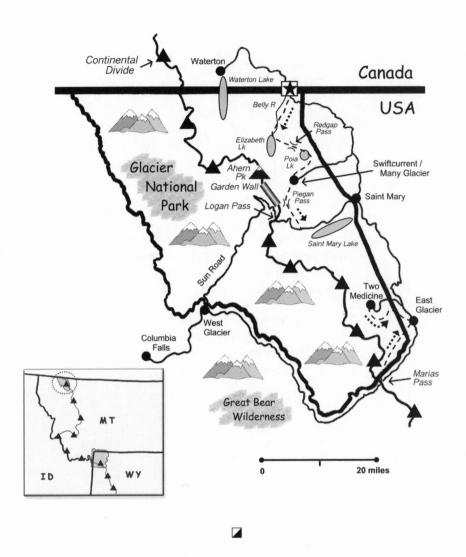

Our hiking route **(Chapters 2 and 3)** from the Canadian border to the Sun Road and from Two
Medicine to Marias Pass, all in Glacier National Park. Our route is shown as a dashed line.
The inset shows the approximate area included in the larger map.

TWO

◪

Ill Wind

Well, you get up in the morning, shake the dew off of your mind,
As the sun pours like honey through the ponderosa pine
You're livin' every moment as if you've just arrived,
Because you know what it means to be alive.

All along the Great Divide,
Yes, we can understand,
What it means to be alive,
All along the Great Divide.

WALKIN' JIM STOLTZ
"All Along the Great Divide"

O N   A   T R A I L near the lake, a hiker appeared. The man struggled to walk, using two hiking staffs to hold himself upright. His arms splayed far apart. His legs swung awkwardly. His feet, cocked at odd angles, thumped with each step. The man's progress was slow and laborious, yet he did make progress.

It was mid-June 1998, exactly a month *before* Kate and the honey blonde bear almost did the do-si-do. The man was walking along Waterton Lake in Alberta, just across the Canadian border from Glacier National Park, Montana. Above him rose the Prince of Wales Hotel, silhouetted at that moment beneath an angry violet sky. Rain poured down. Kate and I stood beneath a shelter, out of sight, and I began to silently weep as I watched the man labor. Kate looked at me quizzically. I hugged

6

her and said that I was just so damn thankful that we had the health to even think about walking the Continental Divide. What God-given privileges we enjoyed: to see, to smell, to walk, to live.

Later we passed the man. He wore a wool shirt, jeans, and stout boots. A grizzled beard shadowed his radiant face. I imagined this city trail along the lake to be the man's wilderness hike. He greeted us heartily, with a great smile, though he never wavered in his progress.

Our own progress toward starting the walk across Montana had slowed considerably. Instead of working on final preparations for departure the following day, Kate and I huddled into our tent and watched a ferocious wind rage off Waterton Lake. The tent sat behind a small building, the only shelter sufficient to keep us from blowing off into the eastern Alberta plains. Two bighorn sheep and a lamb trotted by, pausing in front of the tent to look in. Soft fur covered the lamb, which stood only 18 inches tall. The adults' scraggly appearance foretold the summer heat ahead. But this day summer was on hold. Dark storm clouds hid the peaks; sheets of icy rain raced earthward. We could not see to the far end of the lake where we planned to hike the next day—the initial steps of what we hoped to be 900 miles of walking, the culmination of a year's thought and four solid months of preparation.

A year had passed since Kate and I watched Walkin' Jim Stoltz perform for an environmental conference at the Malheur National Wildlife Refuge in eastern Oregon. Walkin' Jim is a singer-songwriter, a fine photographer, and a long-distance hiker. He travels the country promoting the virtues of wilderness and wild country through his folk music and photography. Jim has walked over 25,000 miles, including the long-distance hiker's "Big Three": the Appalachian Trail (AT), the Pacific Crest Trail (PCT), and the Continental Divide Trail (CDT). Jim is the kind of guy who tells of doing a show in Albuquerque, and then says, "On my walk home to Montana, I . . ." Walkin' Jim inspired us.

Kate and I had been planning a year's leave of absence from work for some time, even before the cancer, though our venue was undecided. After seeing Walkin' Jim's show, we started seriously researching a hike of the CDT. We already knew, of course, that the Continental Divide rises up as the backbone of North America, traversing five states: Montana, Idaho, Wyoming, Colorado, and New Mexico. We knew that the Continental Divide separates the waters of the Pacific from those of the Atlantic. And we knew that the Continental Divide encompasses some of our nation's most dramatic and wild landscapes—rugged granite peaks, lush alpine meadows, and vast high-desert plateaus. What we didn't know then was that in 1978 Congress had designated the CDT as a National Scenic Trail, that the CDT runs roughly 3,100 miles, and that upwards of three-quarters of the trail was complete on the ground, not just in some map-maker's mind. Until listening to Walkin' Jim we also didn't know that each year a handful of people actually walk the entire 3,100 miles in a single backpacking season!

Tackling the challenge of long-distance hiking fit Kate and me well. We'd backpacked extensively for years. We'd once spent most of a year traveling by bicycle. We'd explored rivers by canoe, deep sounds by sea kayak, and quiet mountainsides by cross-country ski. We simply loved, and continue to love, any way of exploring wild country. And whenever that exploration can be formed into a way of life rather than a weekend interlude, all the better. Long-distance hiking fit us like a well-worn boot, with one glaring exception: our anxiety about Kate's health. How would her body react, we wondered, just three years after her final treatments for recurrent cervical cancer?

That anxiety, plus our desire to spend only the three summer months on the trail, led us to temper our approach to the CDT. Soon we began to focus on only the Montana section of the trail, roughly 900 miles from Waterton–Glacier International Peace Park to the Wyoming border just at Yellowstone National Park. Montana was a simple choice—it was my home state, we had been married there, and we longed to move back.

We spent four months in the winter and spring of 1998 preparing for the hike. First, we secured extended leaves of absence from our engineering jobs at Hewlett-Packard Company. Because we are engineers, our second act was to create intricate spreadsheets of everything imaginable: contact names, supply stops, gear weights, elevation profiles, and mean air temperature as a function of moon phase. The gear spreadsheet allowed us to select or omit each carefully weighed item and to move each item between Kate's pack and mine. We plotted overall pack weight and weight within each carefully delineated gear classification on a bar chart—in color with appropriate cross-hatching. For four months before heading to Waterton we packed and unpacked our virtual rucksacks. We weighed and scrutinized and squabbled about gear going into packs that still stood empty. "Hey, what's going on here? I see you slipped the stove into my pack now! What, I suppose you thought I wasn't going to notice?"

Endless planning and data compilation had been a somewhat pitiable attempt to claim control of the hike. Yet we knew that as soon as we pulled on the packs, control was one thing we would largely give up. A fall, a bear, a snowstorm, sickness—the pure, simple stresses of the trail differed so markedly from the artificial, complex stresses of the sterilized working world. Indeed, uncertainties provide the underpinning of any journey—experiencing an unscripted life, feeling the delicious tension of the unknown, and anticipating the satisfaction of successful completion.

Four months of preparation, so much done and still the storm raged across Waterton Lake and still we huddled in the tent. Still we hadn't walked a single step along the CDT.

Now the wind stepped up. Horizontal sheets of rain battered the tent. Kate and I slid deeper into our shared sleeping bag, wondering if June 16 wasn't too early to start a hike from the Canadian border. A low-pressure system sat contentedly atop the Rockies. The low was expected to hold for at least two more days, including the day we were slated to cross Stoney Indian Pass. Stoney Indian, at 6,908 feet, was steep and still snow-covered above 6,200 feet. The next day's forecast called for more snow. No surprise, really—in Kate's and my experience, weather rarely smiles on the start of a long journey.

It poured from 2 A.M. until dawn, with the wind redoubling its efforts of the previous afternoon. The tempest continued as we climbed out of the tent and made for more solid shelter. Shortly we learned that Glacier Park's Going-to-the-Sun Road was newly closed, buried under snow. Later we were somewhat disappointed to learn that we could not buy a pot of tea at the Prince of Wales Hotel. Instead we drank coffee, sat in cushy chairs, and watched whitecaps churn the lake.

The storm continued and soon we agreed to abandon our departure day. I was still in favor of trying Stoney Indian Pass, but Kate favored the safer route up the Belly River, a route that would not take us over any steep, snowy passes. "We haven't done anything stupid yet," she declared to the child in me. "Let's not start now."

◢

That December 1992 day we learned of Kate's cancer I recall as sunny. Strange weather for such a dreary indictment, stranger weather still for our hometown of Corvallis, Oregon, where a cloudless winter day elicits squinty-eyed comments like, "Hey, what's that bright yellow thing in the sky, anyway?"

Everything about that day felt surreal: Kate calling to say the doctor claimed she had cancer, heading to the clinic with racing hearts and hollow stomachs, waiting for the unwanted and unbelievable news while desperately wanting to flee back to the safety of work and our lives.

"I didn't believe that the results were true," Kate has since said. "I thought that when we went in to see the doctor he would say that they had the wrong person. My mind flipped back and forth from not believing it to the panicked feeling of *what if it is really true?*"

And then we heard the words "papillary adenocarcinoma" for the first time and learned that cervical cancer could take Kate's life.

Heading home from the doctor's office, only partway through the workday, we wondered, "Okay, now what? Does this mean we can't ski into the cabin in a few weeks as we'd planned? If Kate has cancer, does she still go to work? Do we cancel our Christmas plans? Do we tell anyone—family, friends, coworkers?" We walked into the house and looked around. A sweater to knit, flies to tie, environmental papers to read, letters to write—in an instant our daily existence became inconsequential. Suddenly we were staring directly into the face of life itself. We sat on the couch, stunned.

How, I wondered, can a person who looks exactly as she did three hours ago, who looks exactly as she did when she ran to work that morning, who could run 20 miles right now at the drop of a hat, who is planning to bicycle around Tasmania in six weeks, *how could that person possibly have cancer?*

*   *   *

In the week after we learned that Kate had cervical adenocarcinoma, we informed our families. The news dampened Christmas celebrations considerably. Prayers at every meal mentioned Kate. Yet there she stood in front of us looking as normal as ever.

Kate had an understandably tough time controlling her thoughts during those days, and was unable to keep from projecting endless unthinkable outcomes. "We went to the play *The Phantom of the Opera*," she recalls. "I can only remember staring at the actors as if I were a thousand miles away, not able to follow the story, caught up in my own worries."

A couple of days after Christmas, Kate and I went cross-country skiing in the North Cascades with several of our dearest friends. We told them about Kate's cancer and about how she was scheduled for cone biopsy surgery as soon as we got back to Corvallis. They expressed shock, but then we all skied through the morning as though nothing was amiss. At lunch, as she sat under snow-covered cedars, Kate's eyes welled up with tears. Heavy snow began to fall. Our friends offered encouragement, but their faces looked troubled. Although it was early in the day, Kate and I turned our skis back downhill—our first steps on a journey we had not chosen, toward an end we did not know.

◪

Though Kate and I expected to average around ten miles per day, we planned to hike short distances in the first days of our walk across Montana. Our change in plans to hiking the CDT's alternate route—up the Belly River instead of over Stoney Indian Pass—meant that our initial hiking days would now be laughably short: six miles the first day, four miles the second. And, not wanting to hurry ourselves, we decided we would take the third day off completely. The slow start would be as much a concession to our minds as our bodies. We hoped to give ourselves time to breathe, time to absorb into the landscape, time to find a new mental space away from home and work.

Kate and I walked across the Canadian border and then to the Belly

River trailhead, near the U.S. Customs house. Within an hour of departing the trailhead, less than three miles into our 900-mile journey, I'd lost my pocketknife and one sole of my four-month-old boots had begun delaminating. I greeted these revelations stoically. Kate had a second knife and I had some duct tape. Besides, wading through ankle-deep mud it was hard to see my boot sole flapping anyway. Four months of preparation and finally the hike was underway!

We had walked this trail to Elizabeth Lake 11 years earlier. Thus the towering mountains and luxuriant valley of the Belly drainage came as a welcome remembrance rather than a surprise. As on that previous trip, Kate and I spent the first night of our CDT hike camped near the Belly River Ranger Station.

We met Marci Johnson that night while we prepared our dinner. Marci wore torn Carhartt jeans. She had a strong laugh and her cheeks glowed. Her work partner, a quiet man, was remarkable because of the roll of barbwire hanging from his pack. The two worked for the U.S. Geological Survey and were taking part in a multiyear grizzly and black bear DNA study.

"Why is the Geological Survey doing fundamental biologic research?" I asked. We were all sitting on logs in the backcountry camp's cooking area. Marci chuckled as if it were a question they often asked themselves and then worked her way through an explanation of the jurisdictional quagmire. We didn't really get it, but Marci's description of the DNA work proved too fascinating for us to spend much time on the peculiar logic of our federal bureaucracy.

It turns out that DNA can be extracted from bear hair follicles and, to a lesser extent, bear scat. The species and sex of a given bear can be identified from that DNA. With appropriate experimental design—mapping the park into grids, randomly sampling from each of these grids, and so on—an accurate estimate of bear population, density, and sex ratio can be made based on hair and scat samples. And all that without direct human-bear interaction or any of those silly-looking radio collars.

The barbwire was used for the hair-sampling portion of study. Marci and her companion were setting two types of hair "traps" for the bears. The first trap rated as pretty low-tech: a short section of barbwire nailed vertically onto a bear scratch tree. Throughout their territory, bears have trees they regularly stop at, gouge with their claws, and rub up against, perhaps for scent-marking. As the bears rub up against the trunk or reach higher to make a mark on the tree, some of their hairs catch on the barbwire. Kate and I had already seen some of these scratch trees along the trail, sometimes with claw marks so high I hoped a stepladder had been involved.

The second style of trap was more elaborate. Marci and her partner constructed barbwire "corrals" in tree stands far away from the trail. They placed a rotting stump in the corral's center and then coated the stump with an odoriferous attractant. Bears had to step over or duck under the wire to access the attractant. Hopefully they would leave hair on the barbwire, or at the stump, which they take some perverse pleasure in rubbing against. Marci spoke with great pride about the attractant, which she had been instrumental in developing. The recipe is a tightly held secret, but Marci hinted that the aromatic blend might include such things as fetid urine, putrid chicken livers, and rotting blood. Imagine building your résumé around that accomplishment.

Marci clearly loved bears. "They're good critters," she said many times as she worked through her explanation of the research. Winding down now, she said, "Hey, have you heard the one about the griz and the priest?" No, in fact, we had not.

Marci's face lit up and she sat forward on her log. "Well, you see, there was this priest. And one Sunday he decided to skip church and go fishin'. He had a fine day on the creek. Walkin' back he ran smack into a grizzly. Quickly he crossed himself and began to pray, 'Dear Lord, please let this bear be a Christian and I'll never skip church again.'

"In front of him the bear drops to its knees, crosses its paws, bows its head, and begins to pray, 'Father in heaven, thank you for this meal which I am about to receive.'"

◪

Kate was in turmoil in the days leading up to the cone biopsy. She had never been a hospital patient before. "I was afraid of how much torture it was going to be," Kate recalls, "IVs, anesthesia, waking up to news of the surgical results." Unfortunately, these were experiences that would soon become all too familiar.

The purpose of the cone biopsy was to remove the small tumor on Kate's cervix, plus enough of the surrounding tissue to hopefully capture all the cancer. The shape of the removed tissue is roughly that of a cone, hence the name "cone biopsy."*

The doctor explained to us that if the pathology report—in other words, the microscopic, cellular study—showed no cancer cells on the edge of the surgically removed tissue, then we were home free. We would go back to our lives and, with the exception of a few more regularly scheduled checkups, we could live like nothing ever happened. If the margins were *not* clear, it meant that the cancer remained and our fight was only starting. The treatment options from mainstream medicine would then be radical hysterectomy—surgical removal of the cervix, uterus, and pelvic lymph nodes—and/or radiation.

We prayed for days, then finally headed to the outpatient wing at our local hospital. Prior to the surgery, the nurses allowed me to stay with Kate after she changed into her hospital gown. I asked them to give Kate some warm blankets when the cold metal of the gurney caused her to shiver. Kate and I didn't talk much. And while she looked scared, I think both of us were feeling a little perturbed that this ordeal had pulled us out of work and the regular schedule of our lives.

I worried throughout the short surgery. Still, I had not overcome the feeling that this couldn't be happening to us, that this whole thing must be a dream. Soon the doctor arrived to tell Giff and Ellen, Kate's parents, and me that the surgery had gone well and that now we would simply wait several days for the pathology report. Kate eventually emerged from the outpatient clinic groggy and sore, but within two days she felt completely normal—so normal that she headed straight back to work.

"Since my project at Hewlett-Packard was on a tight schedule," Kate said later, "my team was expected to go into work during the week between Christmas and New Year's even though the plant was closed. My

---

* A biopsy is any removal of tissue for examination.

boss was sympathetic to my situation, saying, 'Don't come in.' I went to work anyway two days after surgery, not wanting my part of the project to hold up my coworkers."

The wait for the results of the cone biopsy dragged interminably. Waiting is one of cancer treatment's major stresses. Always there are milestones to pass, milestones certain to set the tone for the rest of one's life. This was our first such wait. Giff and Ellen were with us in Corvallis, and Kate and I stayed home from work the day the biopsy results were due, four days after the surgery. When the doctor finally called, the pathology report was not good. Cancer cells showed at the sample margin, meaning the surgery had *not* isolated the cancer. The doctor suggested that Kate have a radical hysterectomy and that the surgery be done in Portland.

By the time Kate hung up the phone, we all knew the results. Our hearts sank and I think we might have all cried. Kate stared at me in disbelief, stunned, and I could only think to hold her and for some reason stammer, "We will not let this change us. We will not go around feeling sorry for ourselves. We will not start acting like we have cancer."

A while later, after some of the emotional trauma had passed, Kate made an appointment with a Portland surgeon, the gynecological oncologist whom our local doctor had recommended for the radical hysterectomy. Then Kate, Giff, Ellen, and I went to the library and checked out every book on cancer we could find. To attack cancer, we knew we had better become well armed; information, in this battle, was armament. I walked around the library with my head spinning, dazed by the enormity of what we were being told threatened Kate's life, yet seeing Kate march through the book stacks as normal to the eye as could be.

◤

After a wet night camped near the Belly River Ranger Station, we packed up and made ready for our second day on the trail. A man and his two boys who had camped across from us were also packing, but they'd decided to head home only one day into their four-day trip. Apparently, the muddy conditions and stomachaches brought on by too much hot chocolate had considerably dampened the boys' enthusiasm. We bid the three of them good hiking, then walked an easy four miles up the valley to Elizabeth Lake, where we looked forward to a day of rest and reflection.

Kate and I spent a good deal of our rest day at the lake simply drinking in the beauty and solitude. At our feet, rounded stones by the thousands colored the lake's edge. Above and around to our right, a sheer face of rock and hidden ledges fell off the side of Natoas Peak. High overhead, mountain goats fearlessly plied the wet rocks. A young goat frolicked like . . . well, like a kid on a playground.

"Billy," I could almost hear mama goat crying, "will you *please* stop doing somersaults next to that 2,000-foot precipice?"

Farther along, at the head of the lake, jagged Ahern Peak leapt skyward, set off by a deep cobalt sky and repeated in the quiet waters before us. Farther around to our left, Redgap Pass showed snow but also bands of crimson rock.

Sandwiched between Redgap Pass and Ahern Peak, a sketchy trail through rock bands traced a path to Ptarmigan Tunnel. The tunnel, built in 1929 and 1930 by the Civilian Conservation Corp, is a hole through an arête, or sharp ridge, known as the Ptarmigan Wall. Before the hole was completed, workers had to climb ropes 120 feet up over the wall, then look down at a 1,000-foot drop to the work zone on the other side. Some didn't have the stomach for it and turned back. Those that stayed to do the difficult, dangerous jackhammering and dynamiting came from solid stock. Most were former hard rock miners from Butte and Idaho.

A backcountry ranger told us the tunnel had just opened for the year, but that a steeply exposed snowfield blocked the trail approach from our side. Given the dangerous snowfield, we decided to forgo hiking through the tunnel and to instead take the route over 7,500-foot Redgap Pass. That ten-mile trip from Elizabeth Lake to Poia Lake—including 2,600 feet of vertical climb to the pass—would serve as our first real hiking test. We had barely walked ten miles total in our first two days coming up the Belly River.

Icy rain pelted down as we departed Elizabeth Lake the next morning. We started into the forest, climbing through bands of rain and mist and clear. Soon we popped out into open country and then onto a snow-covered trail. Thunder sounded near the pass, but low clouds obscured the mountaintops and we could see no lightning.

Remembering a grizzly bear that we had come face-to-face with in this valley 11 years earlier, we sang loudly through much of the climb. We saw no bears this time and I was disappointed, though not deeply.

I fear bears, and mostly here I mean *grizzly* bears. Perhaps "respect" is a better word than "fear," as my anxieties have yet to keep me from voluntary travel in grizzly country. But then again, at night, when the hole in my stomach becomes palpable, "fear" probably is the correct word. At night my overactive imagination often takes charge, refusing the statistical logic that argues the high unlikelihood of bear attack. At night in griz country, my imagination becomes acutely focused on my suddenly diminished stature on the food chain.

Kate suffers no such sleep-depriving malady because of bears. Don't get me wrong—if a grizzly came around the corner, Kate's fear would be as raw as anyone's. Unlike me, however, she will not mentally live through that experience ten times before it happens . . . if it ever does happen.

Friends know about our disparate thoughts on bears. Hence it was me, not Kate, who in the months before the hike received the same e-mail from 40 different people:

> In light of the rising frequency of human/grizzly bear conflicts on the CDT, the Montana Department of Fish, Wildlife, and Parks is advising hikers to take extra precautions and keep alert for bears while on the trail. They advise outdoorsmen to wear noisy little bells so as not to startle bears and to carry pepper spray in case of an encounter with a grizzly. They also advise hikers to know the difference between black bear and grizzly bear scat. Black bear scat is smaller and contains lots of berries and squirrel fur. Grizzly bear scat has little bells in it and smells like pepper.

Ha ha. Ho ho. Very funny.

With no bears and only shallow snow, climbing to Redgap Pass proved remarkably simple. We trudged steeply up for a time, through scarlet bands of rock. I watched Kate for signs of faltering, but she showed none. She marched steadily, breathing easily. Once Kate grimaced against the effort and I quickly asked if everything was okay. She did not reply but instead gave me a look that said, "Why don't you try being someone else's mother for the day?"

Kate felt upset at the weather on that first real hiking test of the journey, nervous about seeing bears, and worried about the lightning. "I thought it would be okay when we got over Redgap Pass," she said later, "but I wasn't sure whether strenuous back-to-back days would be too much for my body. Still, once we got over the top I thought, 'Okay, one pass down, umpteen to go. I'm on my way.'"

The pass proper stood mostly bare of snow. Jagged, sodden peaks still towered above us. We stopped atop the pass to hug, hoot in celebration, and then look ahead. "We're back in the Rockies," I said, a thought that for us meant as much about our joyful state of mind as our geographical location. I was from Montana. Kate and I formed our happy partnership while hiking and skiing in the mountains of Colorado. Suddenly we felt at home again.

We slid down a long snowfield on the backside of the pass and then dropped to tree line as the darkest clouds of the day settled over the ridge tops. Hard, heavy rain started, and soon lightning electrified the pass. Pea-sized hail pounded down for ten minutes. Thunder rocked off the mountainsides. The hail soon changed to rain, then to sunshine, then back to rain, then sunshine again.

We arrived at Poia Lake in six hours, a time identical to that reported by a fit pair of college-aged brothers we met. Our confidence was even further bolstered by the realization that both Kate and I felt able-bodied and well. Though we were soaked, only the mind-numbing "flip-flop, flip-flop" of my delaminated boot had caused us any discomfort all day. Maybe, we dared to hope, this long-distance hiking idea would work. Thank the Lord we successfully completed our first test, I thought. Now if we can only string the days back-to-back like this for three months straight.

◪

A week after learning the cone biopsy results, Kate and I drove up to Portland after work to meet with the surgeon who had been suggested by our local doctor. To our surprise, the surgeon did not examine Kate. He explained that the pathology report now directed Kate's treatment. Kate has since expressed disappointment over the lack of examination. "I thought that someone with such specialized credentials as a 'gynecological oncologist' would want to do an exam and offer more wisdom about my specific case. He only looked at the pathology slides."

The doctor pulled out a photo album and showed us Polaroids of uteruses he had removed. He pointed to the cancerous areas in each and explained that he used the photos to teach medical students. He showed us survival curves for women who had been diagnosed with cervical cancer, then treated via radical hysterectomy. The graphs clearly demonstrated that his results met or beat the national norm, plus that most women who survived for five years postsurgery, survived period. For patients with a tumor of three centimeters or smaller—Kate's was three centimeters—the data showed that 90 percent of those who underwent radical hysterectomy for cervical cancer lived.

Kate surveyed the data with an engineer's eye but thought, "I am not a dot on somebody's chart."

This man was a surgeon, and an excellent one from all indications. Although he was an oncologist with many tools at his disposal, the doctor recommended surgery over radiation treatment and backed up his thoughts by showing us results from comparative studies. He wanted to wait six weeks to allow the cone biopsy to heal. The wait, he explained, would make the radical hysterectomy easier to perform and thus more likely to succeed. Grabbing his calendar, the doctor counted off six weeks and said, "How about February 9? No, no, let's see, I'm at a conference that day. Let's shoot for February 11. Does that work for you?"

I wanted to leave then and there, to escape to somewhere far from the insanity, but Kate calmly said that yes, that would be fine. It felt so strange, scheduling life-saving surgery the way you would a lunch date.

On our way out, the doctor's lead oncology nurse sent us over to look at the hospital wing where Kate would stay after surgery. Because of construction, the darkened ward stood deserted and dusty. It had a dead, dank feel. Our chests constricted. Neither of us felt able to breathe. We held in our emotions for the moment, but later, sitting in the hospital parking garage, Kate cried miserably and I cried, too. We drove home through the night in a cold Oregon rain, crying much of the way. What was happening to us?

Back home that night I tossed and turned in sleeplessness, thoughts tumbling around in my head like clothes in a dryer. In the year leading up to Kate's cervical cancer diagnosis, we had suffered through a number of life's stresses. We had purchased and remodeled our first home, plus Kate had ended one job and started another. Kate had sensed that something was amiss shortly after starting the new job, but she couldn't put her finger on what it was. Several months later, around the time of the cancer diagnosis, Kate was working 12 hours a day, six days a week on a high-profile work project. Perhaps all these stresses combined to weaken Kate's immune system and thus give the cancer a foothold. Perhaps, perhaps not—I realized even then that we would never know.

The following day Kate headed back to work, as she would every day until the radical hysterectomy. She recalls that she used her work as a kind of mental therapy. "When I found out I had cancer, and then that the cone biopsy had not removed it all, I had to tell everyone on my project. They were really supportive of me taking care of myself no matter what. I decided that the best way to pass the six weeks before surgery was to keep working on that stupid project. It was such a mental relief to work on programming and have a whole hour or two where I didn't have that sick, panicky feeling of being suffocated like when I thought about cancer."

While Kate threw herself into her work, I walked around in total detachment, thoroughly unable to concentrate on my job as an environmental engineer. People would yell my name and I would walk obliviously on, separated from the world as if by six inches of Plexiglas.

Only at home did Kate let down her guard. We spent a great deal of time on the couch trying to talk about other things, but we always came back to the cancer. Six weeks is an agonizing amount of time to wait when death's agent has a foothold in your body. There was so much to worry about: Is the cancer growing even now? Will the cancer breach the cervix? Will it metastasize in these 42 days?

I've mentioned that with grizzlies Kate doesn't project fearful thoughts of the future. Waiting for the radical hysterectomy, however, she felt moments of terror. "I did lots of thinking and worrying," Kate remembers. "I teetered between utter disbelief that something lethal could be in my body and abject fear about what lay ahead. I had a hard time ever being happy. I couldn't turn my brain off and I couldn't sleep at night."

I didn't sleep very well during those six weeks either. When we couldn't sleep we read out loud to each other in an effort to take our minds away from the nightmare we were caught up in. We cried often into our pillows. We made a rule that if either of us woke up frightened in the middle of the night, we had to wake the other. The prospect of looking out into the blackness alone, of thinking that this is what death must be like, proved overwhelming. For a time we even slept with a night-light.

THREE

◪

Escape

I learnt a couple of other things from that incident.
I learnt to conserve energy by allowing at least part of myself to believe
I could cope with any emergency. And I realized that this trip was not a game.
There's nothing so real as having to think about survival.

ROBYN DAVIDSON
Tracks

I N J U N E darkness comes late to Glacier National Park. There at Poia
Lake I read by natural light until way past ten, then finally closed my
book and slid deeper into our shared sleeping bag. Kate rolled over
without waking. I couldn't sleep, but instead watched as visions of grizzlies wandered around in my mind.

I remembered the numerous pre-trip warnings Kate's mom, Ellen, had
given us about grizzly danger. Aside from her understandable concern
about Kate's health, grizzlies posed Ellen's major concern about the
Continental Divide hike. "Why can't you just drive along the Divide?"
she asked. "It would be a lot safer."

You have to understand that Chicken Little has nothing over Ellen.
Over the years, every journey we've undertaken has started with Ellen
cataloging the unique and all-too-common manner of death or dismem-
berment we could expect in the region where we would be traveling. She
warned us of banditos in Mexico, killer whales in British Columbia, hurri-
canes in Belize, hepatitis in Costa Rica, and . . . well, you get the idea.

Thus we listened to Ellen with some skepticism when she called a couple of weeks before our departure for Montana and asked, "Did you hear about the man in Glacier Park who got eaten by a grizzly?"

We had not heard.

Now Kate rolled over and wrapped herself around me, momentarily breaking my train of thought. Warming, I unzipped my side of the sleeping bag. I tried to close my mind down for the night but failed, unable to keep from stepping back through the terror that had happened so close by just a few weeks earlier. A 26-year-old Colorado man left home for a summer job driving a tourist bus in Glacier National Park. He arrived early. Few tourists were about. The man wanted to do some exploring and perhaps someone suggested the excellent hikes in the nearby Two Medicine area. Perhaps he heard that the Scenic Point Trail offered great views, so he loaded up a daypack and drove to the trailhead. Possibly he asked others to hike with him but no one was available. Possibly he didn't ask. As he began walking up the trail, the man now fit the profile—young male hiking alone—of the backcountry visitor who most often encounters bear problems.

As the man walked, was he aware? Did he think of bears or did he walk confidently along in the armor of youth? Not two miles up the trail from his car, the man encountered a sow grizzly and two cubs. Perhaps a primordial shiver ran down his spine just before the encounter. Perhaps he simply walked blindly around a corner into the bears. There was undoubtedly a moment of uncertainty for both man and bears, but the stalemate proved overwhelming and the man ran, throwing off his pack. Frantically he left the trail, sprinting downhill across a snowfield. The sow pursued hotly, followed by her eager cubs. Days later the Glacier County coroner pronounced the man's death "due to encounter with an animal, followed by ravage."

Hearing the story had set our emotions on edge. We felt sympathy for the man, his friends—one of whom we talked to in East Glacier—and his family. The incident occurred in mid-May. By early June, around the time Kate and I arrived at Waterton to start our hike, DNA evidence had confirmed that all three bears had fed on the body. Rangers had already killed the sow and one of the cubs, both of which had been found still in the Two Medicine area. The second "cub," a two-year-old, 150-pound male, remained at large.

For Kate and me, the whereabouts of the remaining bear took on special significance. In less than a week we expected to walk along the trail where the man had been killed. On our walks coming into Poia Lake, we had talked about not hiking in the Two Medicine area but then rejected the idea as absurd. The Glacier ecosystem holds hundreds of grizzlies. We obviously would hike near many of them and likely see some of them. Besides, grizzlies can reportedly travel over a hundred miles a day. The young bear would have no home territory and would be nomadic, we reckoned. We were probably as likely to see it near Poia Lake as near Two Medicine. The only way to be certain of not encountering the bear, or any grizzly in Glacier, was not to hike in Glacier, something we were simply unwilling to consider.

I don't know anyone who claims to be unafraid of cancer. I do, however, know several people who claim to be undaunted by grizzlies. Personally, I'd just as soon not have to come face-to-face with either.

Some folks minimize my fear of grizzlies and wave it away with a tougher-than-thou chuckle. I'm not quite sure why those folks consider it uncool to admit being afraid of grizzlies. I'm happy to confess that I have no desire to have a run-in with an angry griz. And I guess I'd like to get something else out right here: *Statistics don't matter.* Terror over a bear attack does not understand percentages or data. Before our hike, I reviewed the stats about the likelihood of a bear attack in Glacier. Sure, more people have been killed this century in Glacier by heart attacks or drowning or vehicle accidents. "But hold on a minute," I thought to myself, "My heart is good, I swim well, and I am not planning on driving through Glacier!"

Fear them or not, grizzly bears and cancer have several things in common. First, they seem to pop up when you least expect them. Second, while the risk of meeting either grizzlies or cancer is low, the consequence can be the loss of one's life. And third—and here is what's truly frightening to most people—*the encounter and what follows can seem wholly uncontrollable.*

I guess the reason I can still hike in grizzly country despite my fear is that I do not believe bear encounters are out of my control. By making noise, learning about bear habits, keeping a clean camp, and doing a hundred other small things, Kate and I could minimize our odds of a sudden encounter with a grizzly. In the same way, by learning about Kate's disease and caring for her mind and body, we stood a fighting chance of beating the cancer.

We choose to be active, not passive, to be participants rather than victims.

◢

The six-week wait for Kate's second surgery, the radical hysterectomy, rushed toward us and at the same time dragged interminably. We spent much of that time seeking second opinions and checking the qualifications of our doctors. We visited or had phone conversations with a half dozen oncologists and had five pathologists review the cone biopsy slides.

We phoned one of those pathologists, Roger Reichert, at his office in St. Louis, Missouri. We had never met Roger, and he knew only two things about us—that we had mutual friends and that I, like him, was brought up in Montana. I broke down into tears as I talked with Roger. He listened kindly and then offered to give us a second opinion on the cone biopsy.

Ten days later, Roger's letter arrived. It began, "Dear Scott and Katie,* It is not as good as we had hoped but not as bad as we had feared. . . ." Roger noted that while the cancer was only superficially invasive into the cervical stroma (the connective tissue layer below the surface), the presence of cancer in some lymphatic channels led him to worry about potential spread of the cancer beyond the cervix. His thoughts on treatment matched with every recommendation we had received from the medical community: hysterectomy with pelvic lymph node dissection.

At our local library, Kate and I checked out books on cancer and found material from the American Cancer Society and the National Cancer Institute. We learned that a simple hysterectomy (removal of the uterus) becomes a radical hysterectomy when the tissues next to the uterus, the

* To the world at large Kate generally goes by "Katie." Only her family and I regularly call her "Kate." She professes no preference; it's just evolved that way over the years.

upper inch or so of the vagina next to the cervix, and the surrounding pelvic lymph nodes and lymph vessels* are removed.

The goal of removing the lymph nodes is to capture any cancer cells that might have migrated into the lymph system from the primary cancer. Once cancer cells get into the lymph system, they can move throughout the body. This movement or spreading of the cancer is termed "metastasis," certainly one of the most frightening words in the English language. As cancer cells begin to spread through the body, the first place they are likely to be caught up is in the lymph nodes nearest the primary cancer. Hence lymph node dissection—i.e., removal—is a major tool for surgeons attacking cancer. The hope is to remove the cancer before it spreads.

Although we were signed up for the surgery, we were not sold on it. Surgery seemed like such a monstrous step; there must be something less invasive available to us, we thought. We had only six weeks to find an alternative, and search we did. At the Oregon Health & Science University Library I entered the keywords "adenocarcinoma + cervical + treatment" and came up with almost a hundred hits in just the three years of literature since 1990. Almost all of the articles concerned surgery, radiation, or chemotherapy—the three big weapons in an oncologist's arsenal. We read the cold, five-year survival rate statistics and wondered how they could apply to Kate. She was still running three or four miles a day and could not fathom the idea of going into the hospital feeling well, then coming out feeling miserable. We read and read and soon chose to focus on only those papers that concluded in statements such as ". . . results in excellent long-term disease-free survival." We looked for alternatives to the radical hysterectomy, researching immunotherapy and cryosurgery and laser surgery and hypothermia and vitamin therapy and nutritional therapy. We asked numerous doctors about these treatments. Everyone pointed us back to radical hysterectomy.

Our research taught us that cervical adenocarcinoma is often thought

---

* Lymph nodes are bean-shaped collections of immune system tissue, connected by lymph vessels (thus looking a bit like a beaded chain). Lymph vessels are not visible to the naked eye, thus surgeons cannot specifically attempt to remove or avoid them. Some lymph vessels are removed along with the nodes during surgery. Removal of nodes and lymph channels can disrupt the flow of lymph through the lymphatic system.

to be more serious than the more common cervical cancer, squamous cell carcinoma. Adenocarcinoma lesions are glandular, while squamous cells arise on the surface of the cervix. Although a Pap smear can detect both types, adenocarcinoma tends to be more difficult to detect and metastasizes (spreads) earlier in its course; thus it has a poorer prognosis. We also learned that the medical profession is no different from any other profession when it comes to jargon—the words sound mysterious at first, but their meanings are really pretty simple. "Papillary" describes the shape of the cancer cells, "adeno" means glandular, and "carcinoma" means a cancerous tumor originating on a membranous free surface.

Finding out just where cervical adenocarcinoma comes from may not be so simple. We soon learned that statistical correlations exist between cervical cancer and age (the average age of women with cervical cancer is between 50 and 55), race and ethnicity (several ethnic groups show higher-than-average cervical cancer incidence), social and economic factors, human papillomavirus (HPV) infection, HIV infection, poor diet, and smoking. Studies also show links between exposure to DES, a compound prescribed to pregnant women to prevent miscarriages between the late 1930s and early 1970s, and clear cell cervical adenocarcinoma.* Some statistical evidence shows that long-term oral contraceptive use may slightly increase the risk of cancer of the cervix, although no definite evidence exists.

Even with all of this information in hand, Kate went through an exceedingly brief "Why me?" phase. She considered the source of the cancer only shortly, then largely discarded the thought. What mattered to us at that point was that *Kate had cancer,* not where it came from.

"When I first found out about the cancer," Kate later told me, "I thought, 'I can't believe it's me.' But I didn't see the purpose of harping on that point. The only way I could think of my situation was to work with it. Either I had to do everything I could to get well, or I had to accept that it was okay for me to go, for my life to end."

Perhaps Kate could focus on what was ahead rather than what was behind because of her pragmatic outlook on life, or perhaps because she is a problem-solver by nature, or perhaps because she sees the victim's

* Although only 1 in 1,000 women whose mothers took DES develop cervical cancer.

role as highly disempowering. Regardless, neither of us could see any value in wasting priceless time and energy in what would be a highly speculative, inconclusive search for the source of Kate's cancer. What mattered at that moment was that Kate had cancer and that we wanted the cancer gone.

Kate was blessed with a new friend during those six weeks of waiting for the radical hysterectomy surgery. Pat Davidson, a friend of a friend, had fought cervical adenocarcinoma several years earlier with surgery, radiation, and chemotherapy. She and her husband, Gary, were still in the process of healing.

Pat and Kate's friendship started with a phone call, then Pat sent a wonderful letter. In it she talked about the medical aspects of cervical cancer. She also included an article detailing the step-by-step procedures of a radical hysterectomy. Most importantly, however, Pat offered her understanding and her experience:

> *I hope you are sleeping well and are able to enjoy aspects of each day. We can't live in the past nor project into the future—we can only live in the now.*
>
> *I found myself at times through the early stages as well as throughout the treatment thinking—or shall I say 'awfulizing'— 'What if it comes back—they didn't get it all'—etc., etc., etc. It's normal and realistic to think of things, but it doesn't have any validity until it's a reality. The old saying, 'Cross that bridge when we get to it' has a lot of bearing. . . .*
>
> *Please know you have a kindred spirit in me and that I am happy to help in any way.*

◪

Our morning at Poia Lake started gloriously. I awoke at 5:30 and emerged from the tent to clear blue sky and sunshine. Kate slept on. I decided to snuggle back in for a few more winks and next woke at 8:45. Perhaps we were a bit tired from that first hiking test, the ten-mile hike over Redgap Pass. Still, as we broke camp for the fifth morning of the hike, there were no sore muscles to report. We walked away from Poia Lake with light hearts, buoyed by the incredible scenery, the warm morning sun, and the recognition that that night we would stay at a cabin near Swiftcurrent Lake and thus have successfully completed the first stage of our walk.

The trail quickly wound down tumultuous Kennedy Creek, then as quickly climbed a forested ridge. We clapped our hands and yelled out. Soon we spotted bear tracks—grizzly tracks—marching down the middle of the trail, and the world took on a new set of possibilities.

We had seen a few single bear tracks while hiking up the Belly River. This was the first continuous bear trail we'd come across, however, and the first to be assuredly a griz. With plenty of mud from the previous day's rain, the tracks showed strong and clear—claws far removed from the toes, pads forming a flattened arc. Claws to heel, the rear print measured roughly ten inches. The bear tracks sat imposingly atop all the hikers' footprints, indicating that the bear had passed this way since the previous afternoon.

Given that it was morning, we were happy to see that the great bear's tracks were heading in the direction we'd just come from, the Poia Lake backcountry camp. This meant, theoretically, that with every step Kate and I were distancing ourselves from whatever waited on the freshest end of those tracks. The tracks told a fascinating story. On steep sections, our bear often slid out in the mud. Elsewhere it walked to the trail's edge and stopped, perhaps to sniff the wind or to look for glacier lilies. Once, rather than walk through a muddy seep, the bear ambled across a long wooden walkway without a hint of pause.

As we pressed on past Ridge Lake, the rocky crags of Cracker Basin began to appear. The trail passed through open meadows lush with wildflowers. We walked comfortably, yelled, clapped hands, and talked happily. Time flowed smoothly, peacefully, until we rounded a corner and started downhill. Suddenly—dead ahead—*grizzly!*

The bear stood broadside, dark and full-bodied against the vibrant green vegetation of the meadow.

"Stop, stop, stop! Grizzly!" I whispered urgently to Kate, though I was sure she saw it at the same moment I did. The bear was 75 yards ahead, staring directly at us.

"Let's go back. Quietly. Turn. Go!" Our words tumbled out in unison.

Moving backward to the corner, I glanced over my shoulder to see if the bear was following us. On my second glance, just as we crested the hill, I saw the bear turn and step out of the meadow and onto the trail, heading in our direction. Now that it was out of the meadow's tall grass, I could see that the bear's legs were dark, its back and shoulders more golden.

"He's coming this way!" I whispered to Kate.

"Shit!"

Crossing into some trees, out of sight from the bear, we took turns urging each other on. "Go! Move! Don't run, but walk fast!"

Kate whispered our escape plan. "Quick, we'll go back a mile to the trail intersection and then go out to the road via the cutoff trail."

A moment later I urged, "Get your bear spray out. Take off the safety." Mine had been out since the second we spotted the grizzly.

"Now?" She looked back skeptically.

"Excuse me, are you saving it for some other time?"

All this as we puffed rapidly up the trail, Kate ahead, me behind, glancing back frequently, seeing nothing but empty trail. Then ten minutes later, as we rounded a corner, I saw a brown movement in some willows, perhaps a hundred yards behind us.

"I see him! He's still coming!"

We pressed on through the next meadow and the next, walking hard, walking together, walking with greater purpose than I ever thought possible. But then on every subsequent corner, our looks back revealed only empty trail. Ten minutes later I said, "It was just a movement in the bush. Maybe it wasn't the bear."

Bear or not, we decided to leave a note at the cutoff trail intersection to warn a group we'd passed earlier in the day, plus any other hikers that might be heading the griz's way. Finally arriving at the intersection, I dropped my pack, pulled out a notebook, and handed it to Kate. I fished out a piece of duct tape and stuck it to the trail sign, while Kate quickly wrote:

12:30 6-21-98 Grizzly bear on trail about 1 mile from here towards Many Glacier. No cubs apparent.

Scott Bischke and Katie Gibson (we took the cutoff trail)

Then, just as Kate moved to post the note, the great bear arrived. Forty yards away, rounding a corner, the bear showed no sign of slowing as it sighted us. Instead, it moved forward with a solid, unhurried pace, head swinging from side to side.

"Bear spray!" I whispered to Kate.

"What about the note?" she had the presence of mind to ask. The bear was now 30 yards and closing.

"Drop it. Let's go!"

We started down the cutoff trail, which left the Poia Lake trail at an acute angle. Thus our retreat momentarily took us closer to the oncoming grizzly. It was a singular moment of great faith that the bear meant us no harm. I followed the griz in my peripheral vision, trying to avoid eye contact. The blur of brown continued as it plodded forward. For one intensely frightening moment I felt certain the bear would make two bounds through the thin vegetation and be upon us. Given the proximity, even a dose of pepper spray seemed unlikely to halt an attack.

Mercifully, the moment passed. The bear continued the last few steps to the sign, and we continued walking down the cutoff trail. I glanced back as our trail dropped over a small lip. The bear stood at the trail intersection sniffing our dropped note.

Over the lip of the hill, the trail plunged down. We walked rapidly. This time I was in front and urged Kate, "Let's go, let's go!"

"I'm all for that," Kate replied.

The trail flattened and we quickly reached another bench. We looked back and saw nothing. Dropping out of the bear's possible line of sight, we decided to jog down the inclines and then walk the flats.

"If we see the bear again," I puffed, "we'll stop, move off the trail, and back up to a tree with our bear sprays held forward."

We recognized two things: that we could not outrun the bear and that this bear was clearly interested, having followed us for over a mile already. I felt glad that despite being filled with adrenalin, we were able to think this clearly, talk to each other, and agree on a course of action.

At another bench top we looked back. Again, no bear. Over the next lip, we jogged again, then walked the next flat, then repeated the process, always glancing back to the top of the previous rise. I held my bear spray in one hand and the notebook, which Kate had handed back to me at some point, in the other. I marveled that she had somehow managed to return the pen to its binder. Fifteen minutes later we heard cars, and soon the trail popped us out directly at the Glacier Park entrance station. Kate pounded on the door, clearly intent on climbing right inside the little booth.

While a line of ten cars waited, we stood outside on the pavement and recounted our story to the ranger. The woman's eyes quickly widened. At the conclusion of our story she thanked us so profusely I surmised that it must get awfully boring handing out brochures all day. Although we were both calmer by then, I noticed Kate's eyes alternately bouncing between the trail and the straight, short path she was maintaining between herself and the door of the entrance booth. For my part, I fumbled for three minutes with the safety on my bear spray, somehow unable to seat it properly.

Kate and I waited for the ranger to call the park's bear biologist, then began the five-mile walk along the pavement to Many Glacier. The first car that passed us sported the vanity license plate GRIZZLY and we laughed, relieved at being, for the moment, on the road. Still, Kate insisted we continue to make noise, arguing that if our bear had only been a mile from the pavement, certainly other bears could be right there at the roadside. And so we walked on and sent out a few yells to dissuade Kate's asphalt-loving bears.

The sudden approach of a park service Suburban, lights flashing, siren wailing, soon checked our progress. The driver pointed to a turnout where we should wait. A moment later the driver climbed from the Suburban, slipped on one of those uncomfortable-looking ranger hats, and introduced himself as Ranger Bob Adams. Ranger Bob was lanky and fit, with solid, bony facial features. He asked us to climb into the Suburban so that he could give us a ride to his office. We explained that we wanted to walk to Many Glacier to maintain the integrity of a continuous CDT hike and that we would stop into his office in a couple of hours, when we arrived there.

"You don't understand," Ranger Bob said. "This is my job. I have to find out about the bear, how it acted, is it one we know about, does the trail need to be shut down, are people on the trail in danger right now. I need the information now, not later."

And so the interview commenced on the side of the road, behind the Suburban, in lightly falling rain. Through questions and our descriptions, Bob quickly established that we could credibly identify a grizzly from a black bear. Then he pulled facts from our rambling story. Most salient to him, it seemed, was that the bear had no cubs, appeared to be in good health, had no distinguishing marks or ear tags or collar, and showed no outward signs of aggression: no bared teeth or chomping or woofing. Bob also keyed in on the fact that though we looked back often, we did not see the bear other than perhaps once.

"That means the bear wasn't chasing you. It was just being curious."

By the time the interview drew to a close, Ranger Bob's small yellow pad curled from the rain. We thanked him for his commitment to safety for both the bears and hikers. He left Grizzly Frequenting signs at nearby trailheads while we continued our walk up the pavement.

An hour later we began to see the buildings of the Many Glacier Hotel nestled on the edge of Swiftcurrent Lake. Past the lodge was the small Swiftcurrent settlement, where we had a cabin reserved for the night.

Then, oddly, the road in front and behind us emptied of cars. Suddenly fifty yards ahead a cinnamon-colored bear stepped out of the bush and onto the asphalt, drawing a muffled, "Oh, shit," from Kate. For a fleeting moment the bear was a grizzly, but then we knew it to be a black bear, and a small one at that. Soon cars approached and the bear disappeared into the brush across the road.

Kate and I started to walk again, both a bit shaky. We finally made it to the hotel at Many Glacier and collapsed into deep chairs in the lobby. Nearby a woman played classical music at the piano while tourists gathered their suitcases and purchased overpriced trinkets. Kate talked excitedly of taking a shower and jumping into clean sheets the minute we got to our cabin and about our planned day of rest. As I listened, I slowly became aware of people all around the lobby staring at us. Following their gazes, I noticed for the first time thick mud tracks making a direct path across the carpet to where we sat.

◤

February 11, 1993. After six long weeks of waiting, the time for Kate's radical hysterectomy finally arrived. We moved into a single room at the hospital in Portland. The construction from a month earlier was complete, and the place didn't feel as frightening. For six weeks now we'd shared the mental agony of waiting. But I could not share, much less relieve, the physical agony of what Kate was about to go through. I could only think of one tiny gesture to make as a show of solidarity—I took a laxative the night before surgery, just like Kate.

We slept together in the hospital bed the night before the radical hysterectomy. At 5 A.M. they woke Kate for an enema, after which she went back to sleep. I could not sleep. The cancer was the grizzly of my dreams, padding around the bed while I lay there with wide, dry eyes.

Later I walked along as the orderly wheeled Kate to the preoperative area. With tears in my eyes I told Kate, "We're going to do well." A surgical nurse tried to reassure me, saying, "Don't worry, we'll take good care of her." Kate lay there without outward emotion and squeezed my hand. In the hall, after they sent me away, I saw our surgeon and said to him, "Do your best." This is our life, I wanted to scream, this is not the time for an off day!

We waited, without word, for three hours—Kate's parents, my parents, and me. Finally, the surgeon burst into the room, full of energy and radiating success. "The surgery went well. There was no sign of cancer in the lymph nodes. Still, we have to wait a week for the pathology report."

We rejoiced and we waited. In a day Kate was walking down the hall, in another day out onto the sky bridge, in still another day across the sky bridge to the VA hospital. I spent each night in the hospital with Kate, and we often worked at stretches and breathing exercises. Flowers and get well cards soon blanketed every open surface in the room.

On the seventh day, we departed the hospital. I took the garden of flowers Kate had received out to the car. Kate struggled to the front door of the Subaru and we slid her into the passenger seat. And then the car would not start—dead battery.

"We've got to push the car to get it started," I said stupidly.

"Don't look at me," came her mordant reply.

Luckily, we were on an incline. I managed to push off and then hop into the car, all without landing on my rear or sending Kate rocketing down the hill driverless.

At home we waited through an interminable week for the pathology report. Cancer discovered in the dissected lymph nodes would mean more treatment—likely radiation or chemotherapy—and would take us a step closer, it seemed, to death. Clear lymph nodes would mean we could go back to our lives minus only the ability to have children. We had, thankfully, discussed having kids just months before the discovery of Kate's cancer and decided no, not us. And so the loss of Kate's ability to bear children was not as upsetting as it could have been. Besides—we always looked for the positive—no more need for birth control!

The day of the phone call finally arrived. We sat on the couch, waiting. I prayed continuously for an hour before the phone appointment. "Please give us our lives back, Lord. . . . Our destiny is plotted; why are we the only two who don't know the direction? Why don't they call?"

Finally the phone rang and time stood still.

Kate and I both grabbed phones and suddenly the doctor was saying, "The pathology report shows no cancer in the lymph nodes." We screamed. The doctor told Kate that with clear nodes she had a 97 percent chance of survival. We hung up and then bear hugged each other until it was hard to breathe. Then we called family and friends, and life felt like a warm sunrise again.

◪

"I *understand* that learning to use the ice axe on the fly is not the preferred method."

I was standing at a pay phone trying to get ice axe lessons from Kate's brother Bill, a true mountaineer. Our full packs sat next to us just outside the restaurant at Swiftcurrent. It was 8 A.M., and we were about to head out for Piegan Pass. Kate and I had never used ice axes, but deep snow reports for Piegan, Pitamakan, and Triple Divide Passes just ahead had convinced us to buy them during our day off. Given that reports had called it a low snow year for Montana as a whole, we had decided to blissfully ignore any need for ice axes during our months of planning for the hike.

I wrapped the strap around my wrist and said, "So repeat that again, how do you hold it? Pick forward or—what did you call it? Adze? Pick forward or adze forward?" On Bill's instruction, I impaled myself in the chest with the shiny adze just as a silver-haired couple passed. The man grabbed the woman's arm and, with a nervous glance back in my direction, urged her in through the door of the restaurant.

A half hour later I breathed a sigh of relief when Kate and I reached the north boat dock of Lake Josephine, the end of the line for most of the tourist hikers we'd been passing. I was happy to have made it that far without eviscerating myself with the ice axe in front of any of them. The tourists come here to ride the boat across the lake for a closer look at Grinnell, The Salamander, and Swiftcurrent Glaciers. These glaciers, like others existing today, are miniscule in comparison to the Ice Age glaciers that helped sculpt Glacier National Park's incredible cirques,* mystical arêtes, and deeply gouged valleys.

Sometimes the tourists get to see more than glaciers, and indeed more than they might want to see. At the backcountry ranger office during our day off, Kate and I had learned that just after the loaded boat pulled away from the south dock days earlier, a grizzly named 007 and his consort emerged from the bush, stepped onto the dock, and proceeded to make noisy bruin whoopee.

Although Grizzly Frequenting signs were posted regularly along the trail, I was happy to see that the south dock stood empty as Kate and I rounded the far end of Lake Josephine and started up Cataract Creek. Just past beautiful Grinnell Lake, a massive rock curtain named The Garden Wall suddenly towered over the trail. Soon Feather Plume Falls rocketed out of the heavens, falling 1,600 feet to the valley floor. Head tilted dumbly skyward, I must have tripped a dozen times as we walked.

Farther on, near broad Morning Eagle Falls, we crossed Cataract Creek in sandals just below where a snowfield covered half the stream.

---

* A deep basin with steep walls.

Shivering, we climbed out of the forested valley, first through low shrubs, then across a grassy alpine zone, and finally into boulders and scree.* Ahead, the clouds began to coalesce into a gray amalgam just below the crest of Cataract Mountain. We crossed a couple of shallow snowfields, but it quickly became apparent that the trail to Piegan Pass was almost entirely clear of snow.

One other thing quickly became apparent as well: Unused ice axes are heavy! By the time we reached Piegan Pass at 7,045 feet, both Kate and I ached. Tired and a bit light-headed, we dropped the packs, sat on the ground, and began to stretch. Behind us The Garden Wall stood rugged and imposing and right at eye level. I felt like a New York City window washer sighting down a long row of skyscrapers.

We didn't sit long as an icy wind started, followed promptly by an icy rain. The trail toward the Sun Road at Siyeh Bend passed alternately between wet, deep snow and wet, deep mud. Soggy feet soon led to blisters and sodden moods for both of us. Pressing on to 10, 11, 12 miles, Kate talked about how she could not do the 15 miles we needed to make our permitted campsite, how this was just too much, how she needed another rest day, and how she wanted to go back to Saint Mary once we hit the Sun Road.

I hurt, too, but I wasn't quite so ready to abandon our hiking permit and find a ride back to Saint Mary for the night. Stepping over an ankle-deep puddle, I said smartly, "It would have been nice if we'd thought of that idea before we started this morning, so that we could have done this section as a day hike and avoided carrying all this weight. Besides, I hate hitchhiking."

Simple ideas stated without malice, I thought as we plodded on through the rain. But like a blind man walking off a cliff, I had just stepped across some inviolate spousal line. Suddenly Kate started to cry wretchedly—tears of salt and soreness and of utter frustration with her unfeeling, good-for-nothing partner. Then came sobs and that anguished look that only accompanies Kate's deepest sadness and anger.

"I'm sorry I didn't know this was going to happen," she yelled at me through cold rain. "But I have to take care of my body, don't I? I have to

---

* A stretch of loose stones.

say when I hurt, right? Didn't we agree to that before the hike started?"

Kate was right. Between the icy rain and my sore muscles, I had lost track of the big picture. I could only answer, "Of course," and then give her a poorly received hug.

At the Sun Road we ended up hitching from Jackson Overlook to Saint Mary, then struggling stiff-legged and sore-footed up the hill to a motel. Stripping off sodden clothes, we found that Kate's legs were heavily swollen, one of the aftereffects of her cancer surgery. Kate stared at her legs in sadness, anger, and frustration. Then she dropped onto the bed, crying miserably.

Just a week into the hike, we lay on the bed in Saint Mary, beaten into submission by blisters and bears, long days and swollen legs, rain and snow and hail. And though we agonized over the decision that night, I think we both knew from the moment we saw Kate's legs that we couldn't go on just then to finish the Glacier Park section of the CDT. We had to go somewhere to the south where we could heal our blisters, hope for better weather, and work up to longer hikes as we walked our way back north to the Sun Road.

Kate lay on the bed in turmoil, eyes puffy. Still fighting the idea of skipping the Glacier Park section for now, Kate sobbed, "I'm sorry I'm not normal anymore."

"I love you," I said, choking up. "You darn well are still normal."

The next day a Browning Police cruiser pulled up on the shoulder of the road, just in front of where Kate and I stood hitchhiking. Sergeant Ralph Hunter stepped out of the squadron car. A big man, he greeted us and asked where we were going. When we told him we were headed from Saint Mary back to our car in East Glacier, he opened the trunk and motioned us to throw our packs in. We climbed into the car, having exchanged only a few words. As he pulled away from the curb, Sergeant Hunter radioed dispatch.

"Yeah, this is Hunter. Got a coupla ten-fourteens out here at the Cut Bank Creek turnoff. Mileage is four-one-nine-two-seven. Out."

As Sergeant Hunter jammed the microphone back into its holder, Kate and I exchanged looks, both of us wondering if "a coupla ten-fourteens" was short for harmless hitchhikers or soon-to-be incarcerated felons. Our worries didn't last long, as Sergeant Hunter soon began peppering us with good-natured questions about our hike.

We told him that we'd decided to change our plans, to head down to East Glacier for a couple of day hikes along the Continental Divide. After that, we planned to drive south to MacDonald Pass near Helena, then hike the CDT back north to Glacier, arriving during the nicer weather of late July. Sergeant Hunter reckoned that our change in plan was not a bad idea. "Weather can get pretty tough around here," he said, "like the winter just passed. We had people shuttling medicine all over the res to folks that were snowed in."

Sergeant Hunter, a Blackfeet Indian, was a long-time veteran of the Blackfeet Police force. He worried aloud a bit about the Blackfeet. "The tribe has a tough time gettin' anything done. We elect a new tribal council every two years, so every time something is just about to get started, we have to start all over. What we need is a few more people on the res with some business sense. Some of our kids get degrees, but if they're successful they usually go somewhere else. We got a pencil factory, wheat farming, and ranching, and that's about it."

As we bounced around a tough corner, Sergeant Hunter told us that he mostly deals with auto accidents. "We got problems with cars hitting cattle on the open range, motorcycles racing down these rotten roads and skidding out. We had a 14-year-old girl killed the other day—that was bad. Biggest problem is drunk drivers. And most folks don't wear their seat belts. Stupid."

Sergeant Hunter dropped us off in East Glacier. Later that afternoon, Kate and I ran into Mel Burchill at the Glacier Park Lodge. Mel was a strong, vibrant woman with ruddy cheeks. We'd met Mel earlier on the bus to Waterton (where we'd started our CDT hike). Mel smiled and laughed warmly as we talked. She spoke of the follies driving a vintage 1930 "Jammer," the open-top, extended-body buses operated in the park. A job driving the Jammers fit Mel well; for nine months of the year she worked as a licensed school bus driver in Cincinnati.

Our banter eventually culminated in Mel's deciding to join Kate and me for a day hike north from Marias Pass to East Glacier. By wearing running shoes and not carrying backpacks, Kate and I could complete more of the CDT while giving the miserable blisters on our feet time to mend. The hike would also give Mel her first chance at seeing Glacier's backcountry. Having only recently arrived in the area, and as yet without hiking partners, she had avoided striking out into bear country alone.

The following morning we parked the car at Marias Pass, near the statue of John F. Stevens. In 1889, James J. Hill, the railroad baron, had charged Stevens with finding the easiest route for Hill's railroad across the Continental Divide. With the help of a Flathead Indian guide named Coonsah, Stevens found the pass in November 1889. At 5,215 feet, Marias Pass met Hill's requirements. It is the lowest crossing of the Continental Divide between Canada and Mexico.

Across the railroad tracks from the Stevens statue, Kate, Mel, and I quickly found the CDT. At Three Bears Lake, not far along, we paused to watch a large bull moose dip its muzzle under the water in search of a meal. Mel chatted excitedly about the moose as we strode on, then laughed when Kate and I began to clap and hoot as we moved farther away from the pass. We told her how we liked to make noise in griz country, to better avoid a sudden encounter that might force a startled bear to quickly make a fight-or-flight decision. Mel looked skeptical. But as we moved deeper into the forest, she soon let out a timid hoot. In another mile, when the trail became scant, Mel sounded off a bit stronger, saying, "Here we come, Mr. Bear." Soon we passed into deep, almost impenetrable bush and Mel sang out, "Hey oh! Hey beeeaaarrrrr!" For the rest of the hike, this became her cry. She belted it out in such a heartfelt, yodeling falsetto that Kate and I referred to her as "The Opera Star" the rest of the day.

Seven hours after starting at Marias Pass, after 14 or 15 miles of mostly forested hiking, the three of us stepped out of the aspens and into Midvale Creek on the edge of East Glacier's golf course. We splashed and frolicked and rejoiced in the cold water on our legs. Mel exuded happiness, thereby doubling our joy at having her along. Across the creek, a golfer looked up from addressing his fairway iron. Happy to see that the ruckus was three sweaty hikers rather than a rambunctious grizzly, the man returned to his game.

The next morning we met Mel for a cinnamon roll at the Two Medicine Grill in East Glacier. She looked fit and happy, only a bit stiff from the previous day's hike. At the counter the headline on someone's *Great Falls Tribune* blared "Killer Grizzly Hunt Restarted." The remaining grizzly from the attack on the Colorado hiker a month earlier, positively identified by an ear tag, had charged a group of 17 hikers the previous day at Two Medicine Lake. Someone at the counter claimed the bear had been shot after press time. No one knew for sure. Kate and I listened to this conversation with intense interest. We had planned another hike without packs that day, this time south from Two Medicine Lake to East Glacier. Our planned route would take us along the trail where the Colorado man had been killed. And now here was that damn grizzly, suddenly appearing again after a month of absence and then immediately deciding to take on an entire herd of humans.

Still, Kate and I wanted to keep progressing along the CDT. Over coffee, we slowly modified our plan, deciding to complete the day's desired section—Two Medicine Lake to East Glacier—on the road rather than on the trail. For all we knew, the griz still haunted the area. A second day without packs, we reckoned, would help our blisters continue to heal. Besides, if we ran the road rather than walking the trail, we would make the 10 or 11 miles in a couple of hours, leaving much of the day to drive south to MacDonald Pass west of Helena. From MacDonald Pass we planned to hike north back to the Going-to-the-Sun Road.

Mel declined our invitation to join in the run, though she graciously shuttled us up to Two Medicine Lake. A cool mist blanketed the hillside, and the two-and-a-half-hour run passed quickly. Twenty-six miles in two days, even without packs, were plenty for Kate and me. Yet we felt stronger and happier and once again hopeful that we might still successfully tackle the entire Montana CDT. Significantly, Mel's positive spirit had buoyed us for two days, at a time when we really needed lifting.

In East Glacier, Kate and I packed our gear during a cold downpour. Dark clouds cloaked the valley, eliminating any hint of Glacier Park's mountains to the west. Weather-wise, our decision to go south looked to be a good one. Mel had agreed to shuttle us to MacDonald Pass near Helena, then return the car to East Glacier after spending the weekend near Missoula with friends. She needed a car, we needed a shuttle. It was an agreement born of convenience.

In four hours we drove down Montana's magnificent Rocky Mountain Front. To walk the same distance—roughly 225 hiking miles from MacDonald Pass back to East Glacier—Kate and I expected to take three weeks, plus a handful of rest days. That was assuming we really could walk ten miles a day, day after day, something we had yet to prove.

The wind howled as we arrived at MacDonald Pass. It was just past sunset, and cold, metal-gray clouds hid the western horizon. Kate and I dumped our gear at a campsite atop the pass, then handed Mel the car keys. Stupid? Sure we'd known Mel for less than 48 hours, but come on, who better to loan your car to than a licensed school bus driver?

Kate and I shivered in the frigid wind while Mel turned the car around. She stopped then and rolled down the window. "Do you want to check and make sure you have everything?" Since it would be three weeks until we'd see the Subaru again, this seemed like a reasonable idea.

The balmy air inside the car warmed my face as I looked around.

"Aren't you freezing? Are you sure you want me to just drive away?" Mel implored as I rifled through boxes.

Yes, we're sure that's really what we want you to do, we said. Again she asked while I considered, then rejected, a down vest. Kate stood aside, huddled against the wind. She was so organized that the concept of having forgotten something didn't even register with her.

"Looks like we got it all," I said and closed the door.

"Are you sure you want me to just drive away?" Mel asked again. Through blue lips, Kate assured her again. Finally we all said, "Be safe," and Mel drove off.

Ten minutes later we had the tent almost up when headlights coming in from the highway signaled the return of the Subaru. The window lowered and Mel's concerned face peered out into the night. "Are you *sure* you want me to just drive away?"

◪

Eight weeks after the radical hysterectomy Kate and I skied in to a Forest Service fire lookout we'd rented in east-central Oregon. Kate felt weak but still wanted to go, so I carried all the gear. We spent the night looking out over the high desert from atop a barren mountain, surrounded by cold air, endless stars, and 360 degrees of glass. Both of us needed that trip to return our spirits to some sort of normalcy.

Five months later we bike toured 800 miles through British Columbia. Kate pedaled solidly, as if the cancer were a thing of distant memory. We had planned to go slowly, and we did, until partway through the trip we realized that in our planning we had neglected to add in a 150-mile stretch of road. Oops! And so instead we biked harder and longer than we had intended.

Life does not always follow the path we foresee.

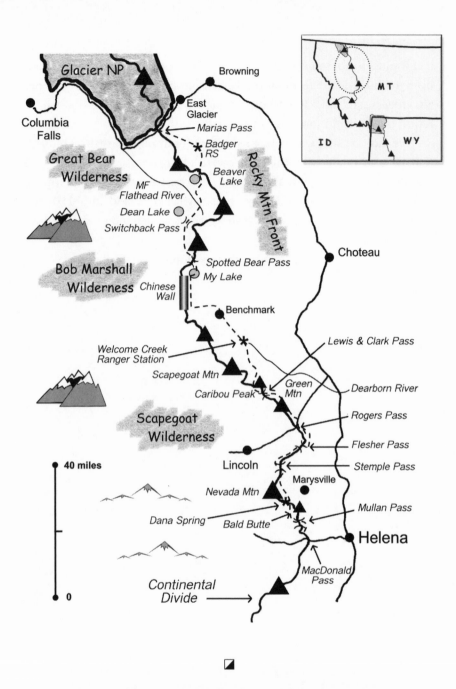

Our hiking route **(Chapters 4, 5, and 6)** from MacDonald Pass near Helena north to
Glacier National Park at Marias Pass. Our route is shown as a dashed line.
The inset shows the approximate area included in the larger map.

FOUR

◪

Climbing the Mountain

Anyone can be a success unless he tries to climb someone else's mountain. The key then is to find your own mountain. Otherwise, you will be competing with people who are not even in your event. . . . A person can be complete or incomplete, but one thing is sure, he cannot be someone else.

DR. GEORGE SHEEHAN
from one of his *Runner's World* essays

K ATE AND I awoke a little disoriented, not sure where we were, then remembered that we had moved south from Glacier Park to MacDonald Pass to get some relief from the cold of Montana's northern mountains. Ah, time for some of that balmy central Montana weather! Doggone it, I thought, maybe I should have left that extra long-sleeved shirt with Mel.

Kate extracted her head from the hot cocoon of the sleeping bag and quickly dove back in. "I can see my breath," she reported. I tentatively stuck a bare arm out into the chill to grab my watch. The watch thermometer read 39 degrees. Outside, the wind whistled, cold wind.

The tent flapped wildly as we moved to break camp. I pulled on every stitch of clothing in my pack, including the long-sleeved shirt, and began to wonder if I needed that vest I'd left behind. Shouldering the packs, Kate and I headed down the pavement toward Helena to the Forest Service road where we would start up the Continental Divide Trail. At the turn we spotted our first CDT "reassurance" symbol. And boy was it

45

reassuring! For the first of what would be a hundred times, one of us shouted excitedly, "We're back on!" True, we'd been hiking "the trail" as recently as the day before in Glacier Park. But Glacier trail signs give no hint that you're walking along the CDT. Suddenly with the reassurance symbol we had community—a transient, ephemeral community, to be sure, but by golly, we thought, other people really do walk along the Divide. And there really *is* a trail. See here, it's even marked!

The sign pointed us north along gravel roads, two miles up to a set of radio towers. Atop the mountain the wind plastered our clothes to our bodies and Kate and I yelled to hear each other. I suppose we couldn't complain; we had moved south for a taste of the tropics and we had found it—a hurricane. Thankfully, on the back side of the mountain the trail, now a jeep road, slipped down through sheltered lodgepole pine for three easy miles to Priest Pass. Valentine Priest, a tuberculosis sufferer from the East who found health in Montana's dry, clean air, built the Priest Pass road in the late 1870s. Priest would have found plenty of clean air this day as wind funneled wildly through the pass. We had to lean into the gale just to stay upright.

Beyond Priest Pass the trail climbed again through open country. In time the cold bite grew less pronounced and I soon unzipped my coat. Overhead, spots of blue showed between the clouds. We hoped that the front was moving past, blowing itself out.

Quickly we dropped back into pine forest and soon into great aspen groves. The wind quieted. For an hour or two we navigated by compass through tall grasses, as no trail existed. Elk droppings littered the ground. A scared deer raced into the trees. The country here was more rounded, softer than the jagged peaks of Glacier. This was a place well suited to crossing the Divide, as John Mullan discovered in the middle 1800s.

Mullan, who had already led a successful party on the Stevens Survey to find a railroad path across the Divide, set his sights on creating a military road across the Northern Rockies. A road across the mountains, tied to the Missouri waterway, would provide a more expedient alternative for shipping troops to the West Coast than an overland crossing of Panama, the current route at the time. Mullan fought for and received $100,000 from Congress to build the road between Fort Benton, Montana, and Fort Walla Walla, Washington, a distance of 624 miles. The Mullan Road was started in June 1859 and was completed slightly over three years later. I've had street projects in my neighborhood take longer than that.

Today a railroad tunnel runs under the dry saddle at Mullan Pass for trains heading east into and west out of Helena. As Kate and I walked above the tunnel, a train passed beneath us. We followed the train across the pass and then decided to make camp on an open hillside above the tracks. We had barely hiked seven miles for the day. Still, we were carrying heavy packs, plus nursing abused feet that had covered 26 miles in the previous two days. Kate set up the tent at the forest's edge while I headed down to pump and purify water near the tunnel's east portal.

By the time I returned, the clouds had blown themselves out. Blue dominated the sky. Kate sat in front of the tent, intoxicated by the sun's warmth, brewing coffee. She had happily discovered another CDT symbol just behind our camp. Indian paintbrush, shooting stars, and a bouquet of other wildflowers dappled the ground. To the east sat Helena, and beyond that the Big Belt Mountains. We sat for several hours, reading to each other, drinking coffee, preparing dinner, and enjoying the sun.

For the first time on the hike, we felt totally relaxed. No mud or wind or wet or cold or snowy passes. And no grizzlies. Our feet even felt a bit better. The blisters had started healing, helped immensely by a day or two of being dry. Also, during our days around East Glacier I had picked up a new pair of boots, so we no longer had to listen to the incessant "flip-flop, flip-flop" of my unattached sole.

Dusk settled. Stars appeared. A glow from the lights of Helena began to show to the east. From below came the clatter of steel on steel, at first faint, then louder, and then louder yet. Suddenly a shrill horn joined the metallic din and we imagined this otherworldly cacophony to be a spaceship approaching from some distant supernova. The clatter climbed to a crescendo, then slowly began to dissipate as the mother ship was swallowed, car by car, into the black hole of the mountain.

◢

By four months after the radical hysterectomy, June 1993, our lives had returned to near their normal pattern. We fished, hiked, and canoed through the first summer. Two friends, Ed and Colleen Llewellyn, introduced us to sea kayaking, though our first kayaking trip was down the Columbia River. Kate also biked through the Gulf Islands of British Columbia on a secretive "women only" trip. She never would tell me much about that trip, never would tell me if she and her friends had danced around the fire, beating their bare chests while intoning some primitive chant. I admit suspicion, however, as I have since seen a photo showing several of the women mouthing fat cigars.

In October 1993, eight months after the radical hysterectomy, Kate ran the Victoria Marathon. Twenty-six miles, 385 yards. Kate had returned to running with great happiness, in a manner wholly slanted toward making her feel as though the cancer and the surgery had not changed her.

At work, Kate's new project took her to Switzerland for a short time.

During those months, Kate went through regular checkups with her Corvallis gynecologist. He noted a "nodule" at her three- and six-month postoperative checkups and a "lesion" at her ten-month checkup. He declared them to be "innocent" and told us not to be concerned. "I believed him," Kate remembers. "I *wanted* to believe him."

Another more subtle issue began to express itself about ten months after the radical hysterectomy: Kate's thighs began to swell. It would be two years before we would truly understand the ramifications of what was happening, a malady of the lymphatic system called "lymphedema."

Lymph is the body's magic elixir of proteins and white blood cells. Lymph harbors some of the body's immune system, its defense against disease. Lymph travels away from the heart in the bloodstream. On the return journey, however, it moves through a separate network of vessels, the lymphatic system, which includes no pump counterpart to the heart. Instead, lymph moves back to the heart by the repetitive squeeze of muscle fiber. Lymphatic vessels pass through nodes—literally collection points—on their way back to the heart. Obstructed nodes or surgical removal of these nodes can lead to swelling—in medical terms, lymphedema.

Prior to the radical hysterectomy, our Portland surgical oncologist mentioned that in a few cases the surgery could cause leg swelling. He added that if it happens, women simply wear compression stockings to combat the swelling. No problem, apparently; nothing more was mentioned.

I will repeat a bit of what I wrote earlier, since lymph and lymph flow are such an integral part of this story. As cancer cells move away from the primary cancer site, they are likely to be caught up in the lymph nodes. It is these nodes that surgeons remove in hopes of catching any cancer cells before they begin to move around the body (i.e., to metastasize). During the radical hysterectomy, our Portland surgical oncologist removed 30 of Kate's pelvic lymph nodes. People have different numbers of lymph nodes in a given location. The doctor felt confident that 30 lymph nodes represented a large percentage of those available in Kate's pelvic area. Thankfully, the pathology reports on the nodes proved negative. Ten months later, Kate's legs began to swell because the lymph no longer had free passage out of her legs. Delayed swelling like Kate's, we learned much later, can be a sign of a low-grade infection, or worse, recurrent cancer.

The leg swelling came and went over the months and we didn't grow overly concerned about it. But at 14 months postsurgery we did find reason for grave concern. At a checkup in Corvallis, our doctor found that a mobile, golf-ball-sized growth had formed along Kate's vaginal wall. Consultations in Corvallis and with our Portland doctor confirmed that this growth was almost certainly a lymphocyst, a nonmalignant pooling of lymph fluid that could be safely drained. Lymphocysts following lymph node removal, the Portland doctor explained, are not unusual given the interrupted lymph flow path. Using ultrasound to guide him, our Corvallis doctor drained much of the fluid from the cyst with a long, frightening needle. Kate anxiously waited for the pathology results the following week while at the job site in Switzerland. Though the cyst remained, fortunately the tests on the fluid proved—as expected—negative for cancer.

Four months later, in August 1994—18 months post–radical hysterectomy—the cyst had expanded to the size of a tennis ball. Our doctors' collective medical opinion was that we should simply continue to monitor the cyst rather than intervene. Three weeks later the cyst burst, causing Kate to race home from work.

Kate recalls feeling awe at that moment of the fragility of life. "When the cyst burst I was taking a training class at work. Suddenly everything changed, and I was calling our Portland doctor about the fluid running down my legs and trying to decide how serious it was. In regular life we don't regard how many things, many that we don't understand, have to go right for us every day just to live. We rely on so many fragile systems unappreciatively."

Our Corvallis doctor was away, but his partner told us that as long as Kate wasn't showing any sign of fever or infection, we should just continue to monitor the situation. In the days ahead, Kate's regular doctors concurred. They were not concerned enough to advise Kate and me to change our plans for sea kayaking down the Stikine River in western British Columbia and southeast Alaska. They said we could put off any further testing until we returned home. It was a remote, nine-day trip, and even though the lymphocyst continued to drain every day, Kate felt adamant that we go.

"I wanted to go to the Stikine that September," Kate told me later, "because I remembered from the radical hysterectomy how slow everything with doctors, tests, and surgeries goes. I pictured sitting and waiting for test results for a week versus going on a great trip. I voted for the trip. I figured that if something serious was wrong with me, I wanted to do something fun before dealing with it. I thought the Stikine would be an awesome wilderness experience and I really wanted to go. Later, when things looked really bad, it was a great escape from reality to remember flying in to Telegraph Creek, putting together our foldable sea kayak, and then floating it down the big river with the monster logs, seals, salmon, glaciers, and bear prints everywhere."

A week after we returned from the Stikine, an examination by Kate's local doctor incredibly revealed a firm, fixed, baseball-size lesion on Kate's left pelvic sidewall. Though impressed that the cyst seemed fixed rather than movable, our Portland doctor did not express alarm during a phone consultation. He assured our local doctor and us that it was still more likely that the lesion was a benign lymphocyst than a cancerous tumor. Nonetheless, the Portland doctor requested a CAT scan be taken and the results sent up to him. A week later he called Kate at work to say that the CAT scan had revealed a thick-walled, complex mass that did not appear simply fluid-filled. "My best guess now," he told her, "is that the lesion is cancerous. I think we need to do surgery to remove it."

After Kate hung up, she quickly phoned me. We both left work for the day and walked home. Once there, we went for a run and did household chores, but with our minds racing through a million thoughts. They can't know, we kept assuring each other; they won't know if it's cancerous without a biopsy. We have hope, we thought. We must hope that the interpretation of the CAT scan was wrong.

◪

For the first time during our hike along the Divide, we awoke to blue sky and a dry tent. Ten minutes of walking brought us to the Mullan Road, where Kate complained that her feet ached miserably from blisters. I had already taken all the food, but I wondered if I might get a sufficiently large pack to carry everything. It was a silly thought, and when I mentioned it aloud to Kate, she gave me a cool look that needed no accompanying words.

Atop the next hill, we had to make a decision: Attempt to stay directly along the crest of the Divide, over Greenhorn Mountain, or follow roads just below the crest. The rounded crest ahead did not look particularly strenuous. Still, we had read that the trail was not complete here and that this "official" route entailed quite a bit of bushwhacking. Kate made an impassioned plea for the stable tread of the roads. We were only a couple of miles into the day, yet it was apparent that her feet were causing her great pain.

"I can hear dread in your voice," I told her. "And I can see clouds in your eyes. Are you sure we shouldn't just consider quitting the hike altogether?"

"I just need a rest day, okay?" Kate replied with fervor. "Then I'll be fine." If we take a rest day now, I thought, the blisters should almost surely be healed by the time we start up again. Then, by the time we reach Stemple Pass in a couple of days, we should finally know if this dream of walking the Divide has been ill conceived from the start.

And so we stopped along Dog Creek after putting in only six or seven

miles for the day. Nearby we found a beat-up cabin, apparently abandoned, its door ajar. The rubble of a disorganized life—rotting woodpiles,
old wire spools, holey buckets, rusted pipes—littered the forest around
the cabin. We ate lunch on the porch, then pushed the door open. Inside
was more chaos—torn mattresses, yellowed newspapers, broken chairs
and tables, old bottles, garbage. Yet amidst the debris several new packages of Ramen noodles sat on a shelf next to a few newish pots and pans.
We considered, just briefly, staying in the cabin. Then Kate reminded me
that Ted Kaczynski, the "Unabomber," had lived a mere 20 miles from
there, near Stemple Pass. We contemplated the likelihood of Ted having
friends in the neighborhood. All things considered, we decided, we
should probably find a place to camp farther up the creek.

A half mile on, Kate opted to rest while I set up the tent and then
climbed nearby Bald Butte. Mining ruins and test pits littered the hillsides. For a time in the mid and late 1800s, this area was one of the
hotbeds of Montana's hard rock mining era. From Bannack to Virginia
City to Helena men cut into the hillsides, driven by gold fever.
Marysville, just a couple of miles from Bald Butte, once teemed with several thousand people. Its economic foundation, the Drum Lummon
Mine, produced an estimated $50,000,000 in gold. Now Marysville is
largely a ghost town, although it has one fancy restaurant, a small ski hill,
and a scattering of homes.

I sat on a rock outcrop atop Bald Butte and gazed up at an endless blue
dome. Montana's clichéd trademark "Big Sky" is all too true. To the west
loomed Black and Nevada Mountains. To the southwest rose the snow-
covered peaks of the Pintlers. Southeast stood Greenhorn Mountain,
more easterly Helena and the Big Belts, and a little farther north the Gates
of the Mountains Wilderness. Billowy clouds enhanced the illusion of
looking off into eternity. From that trifling little peak in the middle of
what many might consider lackluster Helena National Forest, I could see
to forever. And what I saw felt right: dry lands, big rivers, distant peaks,
vast open spaces. We will live in Montana again soon, I promised myself.

When I returned to the tent, I found Kate stretched out, fast asleep.
Her feet dangled in Dog Creek where earlier she'd been freezing her agonizing blisters. I stood there looking at her in amazement. No one else

sees the troubles Kate suffers: living with a radiation-hardened bladder that sometimes leaks, that holds so little volume that she has to pee 20 times a day and has to get up two, three, four times a night; living with swelling legs, pulling on tight compression stockings even in the hottest weather; living with a radiation-damaged bowel, sometimes uncontrollable diarrhea, an acidic system, and dietary limits—nothing spicy, no lactose; living with the indignity of taking so many pills—pain pills, estrogen, vitamins, antidiarrheals.

Yet always Kate finds a way to cope and, even more importantly, a way to excel.

So much has changed because of the cancer and the cancer treatment. But what hasn't changed is Kate's spirit. As I stood there she groggily awoke, then pulled her feet quickly out of the creek. "Ouch! My feet are numb! I must have fallen asleep." Kate rubbed her feet vigorously and then said with a smile, "Ah, but at least they feel better."

From her creekside sleeping spot, Kate stumbled upstream to the edge of a clear-cut where we would make dinner. Small golden stoneflies fluttered in the air above us, disproportionate in number to the size of the tiny stream. Kate played beautiful flute music as the sun began to set over Roundtop Mountain. Putting the small wooden instrument down, she said greedily, "When I get to Lincoln, I'm heading straight for a three-pancake breakfast, topped with bananas and walnuts. And you know what else?"

We both knew that Kate had already described three times what she would eat, never mind that she couldn't eat the dairy products in the pancakes. But with that infectious smile, I had to play along.

"What?" I asked.

"A big plate of hash browns!" Kate spouted triumphantly. Now two weeks and almost a hundred miles out on the trail, her hiker's hunger was beginning to kick in.

◪

October 5, 1994. The day before Kate's third surgery—the one to remove potentially recurrent cancer—we rose late, then went for our favorite run.

We bought three papers, brewed two pots of tea, and latched onto our morning as though we would never let it go. That afternoon we drove to the hospital in Portland so Kate could have her blood drawn and we could meet with our doctor prior to checking in the next day. While doing some paperwork, we talked with a nurse we recognized from Kate's radical hysterectomy surgery 20 months earlier. The nurse did not remember us. She asked about the New Zealand emblem on my shirt, then mentioned something about hiking, and seemed unaware of Kate's upcoming surgery. I am continually stunned at how a hospital works. People go on with their day-to-day tasks, chatting and laughing while others weave through the same tapestry on their own life-and-death march. Somehow in the hospital the two threads plait into an uneasy reality.

The blood draw did not go well. The tech tried repeatedly to insert a needle into one of Kate's hidden veins. By the time he finally found a usable vessel, Kate looked woozy. "Keep breathing," I urged her, but suddenly her head fell between her legs and she would not respond. As I tried to hold Kate up, the tech struggled to extract the needle from her arm. It was 30 minutes before we could warm her up enough to find another usable vein.

Later in the day, our Portland surgical oncologist and his students met us in a small conference room where they presented Kate's recent CAT scans. Each slice showed another stacked cross-section of the abdomen. The growth was readily visible, with a slightly clouded interior. Our doctor explained that we could do nothing and hope that the mass was a lymphocyst, or we could surgically biopsy the mass to determine if it was malignant. He recommended the latter approach.

Our doctor knew that in the past week we had sought out second opinions from numerous oncologists around the Pacific Northwest. He appeared visibly pleased that no one had contradicted his treatment plan—that the other oncologists had supported everything he had told us. We asked our doctor a long list of questions about the options and the proposed procedure, which he answered precisely. We also asked if he could use the omentum to help Kate's reduced lymphatic flow. This was a procedure we'd recently read about. His answer was not encouraging.

Then he asked one of his students to describe the omentum—a fold in the abdominal membrane—and the student answered incorrectly.

I pooped my pants the following morning. Like Kate, I had taken a laxative the previous evening, wanting to show my support and share in the tiniest way the physical agony she would experience because of the surgery. We had stayed in a nice apartment in Portland with Kate's parents, Giff and Ellen. We rented a movie to pass the evening, somehow selecting a comedy whose lone tragedy was that a woman dies of cancer. Kate didn't cry, but when Ellen said, "Let's not watch the end of this, okay?" Kate didn't argue. We slept pretty well, surprisingly well given the JELL-O and laxative diet. Early in the morning Ellen woke Kate and quietly helped her with an enema.

As we departed for the hospital, already late, I hid from Giff and Ellen so they wouldn't see my soiled pants. Kate drove while I changed clothes in the car. Several times I wanted to say things about her driving in the congested traffic, and then realized how ridiculous my thoughts were relative to the surgery she would undergo that day. Mostly we drove in silence. Kate's demeanor was pragmatic. During the week since we'd scheduled the surgery, she'd expressed worry and apprehension. Now with the decision made and the task at hand, Kate seemed outwardly strong, her focus fully on getting ready for surgery.

Arriving at the hospital, we were greeted on our floor, 5C, by another nurse we remembered, this time one who remembered us. "What are *you* doing back here?" she asked Kate. Kate's chest constricted while I stumbled through an answer. Even with her pragmatic approach, Kate's emotions lay just below the surface. The moment the door to our room closed behind the nurse, Kate burst into tears.

We had a roommate this time, Elaine. She returned from a walk shortly after Kate changed into a hospital gown. Elaine looked like an Auschwitz prisoner: bones tight under the skin, eyes sunken, hair threadbare and wispy. Seeing Elaine rocketed me back into the reality of 5C, the cancer ward. As with our previous trip to the hospital—for Kate's radical hysterectomy—I wondered why the cancer ward had been located in "the big C" wing. And I flashed back to the beautiful woman who had been in the room next to us during that stay. She had peacefully died of cancer during the night while we slept. In the morning her room stood empty and sanitized. The woman had been 28. Kate this day was 31. So many times in the past 20 months I reflected on how that scenario could have nothing to do with us. And now here stood Elaine with her sunken face and Kate with her vibrancy and beautiful hair. It was as though we were being forced to join a fraternity that we didn't want to be in. I felt ready to vomit.

Elaine asked too many questions, most of which Kate evaded. Soon Loreena, another nurse we remembered and liked, stuck her head in the door. She greeted us warmly and then said, "They're calling for you." Loreena's words brought agony, though Kate's facial expressions gave no indication of her inward emotions.

"I was feeling dread," Kate remembers. "But also I was just anxious to get the whole thing over with."

Kate climbed onto the gurney and off we went. The orderly raced down the hall so fast I could barely keep up. One of the pre-op nurses engaged Kate in some friendly talk about running as she readied Kate for surgery. When the anesthesiologist arrived to take Kate away, the nurse sternly insisted that he do a good job with Kate. I said goodbye to Kate and the nurse squeezed my arm. Downstairs, outside the waiting room, I ran into our doctor. Just as at the previous surgery, I told him to do his best. "Sure, of course," he answered and disappeared.

The surgery started at 12:45. By 3:00 we'd heard no word, although they had said they'd call out periodically. Giff and Ellen read. . . . I prayed continuously for four hours. . . . I had worn my luckiest shirt. . . . Finally our doctor arrived at the waiting room with his chief oncology nurse. They closed the door, not making eye contact, and suddenly I knew something was wrong with the universe.

"More adenocarcinoma. We were unable to remove it all."

I nearly fainted. The oncology nurse suggested that we all go upstairs to the doctor's office. They pointed us in that direction and I cried all the way. When we sat and talked further, I had to kneel on the floor because I again felt faint. They told us that not all the cancer could be removed and that the tumor had grown dangerously close to Kate's bladder and ureters and that they had found another point near her backbone.

Ellen asked most of the questions. She asked about a possible correlation between the cancer and Kate's work in front of a computer screen and about proper care for sick patients and about treatment at Sloan-Kettering. And she told them she didn't care one lick about stepping on anyone's toes in order to get her daughter the best possible treatment.

And after long minutes of questioning, Ellen finally asked, "So what we're saying here is that Kate has terminal cancer. Am I right?"

Neither the doctor nor his nurse said no. Then the talk turned to how long Kate had left to live and medical choices and quality of life. Listening back and forth, I felt ready to explode. Finally I burst out saying that I could not—that *we* could not—continue this conversation without Kate.

Somewhere in the middle of it all, the doctor said, "You should be prepared for the fact that Katie might not be around next summer." Summer was only eight months away! His nurse added, "We consider the hospital a terrible place to die."

When we finished talking, the nurse made a phone call and learned that Kate was already out of the recovery room, heading back to a private room they had found for her. We arrived there just as Kate did. She lay on the gurney outside the room, still heavily anesthetized but able to recognize us. I followed as the orderlies wheeled her inside. As they lifted her to the bed, Kate kept looking at me, fearful, wide-eyed, demanding and—anesthesia or not—I knew my eyes hid nothing from her.

When I could finally go near she whispered thickly, "How did we do?" and I could only say, "We didn't do very well, buddy."

I brushed my hands through her hair. I was crying silently, and all I could see in Kate's eyes was a clouded yet clear sadness in what I had just told her.

◪

In two days Kate and I hiked 20 miles through Helena National Forest, from Dog Creek to Stemple Pass. In those days we saw a cross-section of the "multiple use" demands mankind puts on our national forests. Industrial logging, for example, has scarred the landscape. In the valleys on both sides of the Divide, clear-cuts have turned the forest into an ugly patchwork of tortured ground and slash piles interspersed with fragments of forest. A friend once swore he had never seen worse logging devastation than he witnessed while walking in the Helena National Forest.

Mining has also left its scars. We passed numerous digs, all inactive. Most, I assume, were failures of the late 1800s, though not for lack of optimism on the part of the hard rock miners. Names like "Hope Creek" and "Faith Gulch" reflect great expectations. Lack of success didn't mean lack of work, however, based on the tons of rock and dirt these men moved, all by pick, shovel, and cart. Once we crawled into a mine shaft that dove deep into the mountainside. Cart tracks sliced back into the narrow cavity, diminishing into the darkness, then disappearing into the inky black water that filled the descending tunnel. These open cavities in the hillsides provide a ready avenue for acid mine drainage. In many places orange rivulets stained the land.

Old mining scars have been joined by a new blemish on the landscape: off-highway vehicle (OHV) tracks. According to the map, no road exists between Black Mountain and Nevada Mountain, and also no road for miles north of that. With the advent of OHVs—and here I mean sport utility vehicles, motorcycles, and especially the four-wheel, fat-tire motor scooters—there is often no longer an "end" to the road. A rutted double track pushes far up the south side of Black Mountain. Another has been created out of the single track up the east and north sides of Nevada Mountain. Sadly, even in places that still seem pristine one often comes across a faint OHV track, an indication that the land's defenses have been compromised.

South of Stemple Pass, two couples on four fat-tired OHVs came racing down the trail toward us. All four wore cowboy hats. We heard the roar of the engines five minutes before we saw the group. They raced past, waving happily to us, hooting and hollering. There could be no doubt they were having a good time. But just because something is fun, I wondered as they passed, is it also right? Is it appropriate?

Possibly these men and women with their cowboy hats were ranchers. Far down off the Divide, Kate and I frequently saw grazing cattle, another challenge to the land. As is true with forestry and mining and OHVs, the stresses the cattle industry puts on public lands are well documented, from overgrazing to riparian zone destruction to taxpayer subsidization. Still, the historical use of public lands for livestock grazing is so ingrained here that it is often claimed as a right rather than a privilege. The mystique of the cowboy still permeates Montana culture.

Nonmotorized recreationalists such as hikers, horsemen, and bicyclists also add to stress on the environment, with fire and footprints and overuse. Kate and I saw two bikers on this section of the trail. The two were traveling The Great Divide Route, a bicycle route that follows mostly gravel roads paralleling the Continental Divide. The bicycle route and hiker's routes don't often coincide, except at places where the CDT rolls along a road on a ridge top.

Multiple use is a drama of demands on the land that often pits user groups against each other. The drama centers on how man can slice up the commons into pieces big enough for everyone. In this drama the land becomes secondary to the personalities and self-interests of the people. The land is seen to have value only as it benefits man. But another view exists: Aldo Leopold—one of the founding fathers of The Wilderness Society—taught us that in a land ethic, the land, its soils, water, plants, and animals are recognized to have value outside the framework of man. What's still amazing, Leopold taught, what's still so magical, what we should begin focusing on, is the land itself.

Kate walked stronger during those 20 miles between Dog Creek and Stemple Pass, the blister crisis apparently over. As our blisters disappeared, our morale reappeared. When we saw CDT reassurance signs, together we yelled out, "We're back on!" Kate's spirits, so tied to her physical well-being, soared. On rugged climbs, her talk was peppered with phrases like, "This won't be so bad," or, happily, "That was a tough one, huh?" At the crest of Black Mountain, Kate danced a jig.

We saw only three groups in two days as we walked from Bald Butte to Stemple Pass. Even surrounded by so many reminders of man's demands on the landscape, for hours on end we hiked alone, feeling the land's enchantment. We walked in a silence broken only by the wind, absorbing the power of the sun and the mysticism of the forest. North of Nevada Mountain we crossed several incredible saddles—massive, broad, and barren, land bridges dropping into steep, U-shaped valleys that were often covered in a dazzling green carpet of pines. Wind pushed our hair and ahead the uplifted spine of the Divide showed for miles. We marveled at the flowers blanketing the hillsides and when finally I could stand it no more I burst into song: "The hills are alive with the sound of music. . . ." No one heard but Kate, and she turned back to give me a mirthful look. We felt so very lucky to be alive. Now, I thought, if we just have the strength to keep walking mile by mile, day by day.

We spent a rest day camped near Dana Springs, partway to Stemple Pass. Here was ready water and a fine view southwest to the Flint Range. Here was a place where we could recuperate and reflect on the first weeks of our long-distance hike. One evening we sat in deep grass near the spring, watching a disappearing sun color the sky, feeling the gentle wind, and talking. With the day off to rest and think, I asked Kate, "The question becomes, are we enjoying this? And more important, is the hike putting your health at risk?"

For Kate, life is most often lived in the moment. Rarely does she have haunting memories of yesterday's digressions or take fearful looks into tomorrow. Today. Now. Comfortable and happy there in the grass, Kate barely acknowledged my questions. Yes, she was fine. This is what we're here for, isn't it? This very sunset, the feel of this blade of grass, the open space all around us. We sat quietly for a while, with Kate lying belly down in the field, face in the grass.

Soon, without looking up, she murmured, "This is a bug's-eye view. If you're a bug, your whole world is grass." And how true. When you crawl along the ground, it's hard to see beyond the blades of grass, but open your wings to the sky, and suddenly the world transforms.

◪

Kate slid in and out of a postoperative stupor through most of the evening following the discovery of her cancer recurrence. She slept in two-hour intervals, waking whenever a nurse came in to take her vital signs. Much of the night we slept holding hands. When she woke, we looked at each other and my heart broke.

Sometime in the darkness of early morning Kate's eyes opened and showed clear. We looked at the stars through her windows. I worried that because of her postsurgery grogginess she might not have remembered that the cancer remained. It was a reality I knew she would not want me to withhold from her, even so soon after surgery. When I asked if she recalled what I told her when she returned to the room, she said yes, and her eyes filled with tears.

"Please, let's not talk about it right now," Kate whispered hoarsely. "I can't think about that right now. Tell me about something happy. Tell me about the Stikine. Please tell me something happy." And so I told her about our new sea kayak—*Chile Roja*—and about our trip down the Stikine, and she smiled just a bit before slipping back to sleep.

More family besides Kate's folks began to arrive the day after the surgery. My sister and brother-in-law, Suz and Dennis, showed up first. They were on their way to the marathon in Victoria, British Columbia, a marathon Kate and I had been training for just a month earlier. Kate said she did not want visitors, so I went to the cafeteria with them. We cried, held hands, and hugged. I felt so useless to Kate, so helpless to change anything, but then Dennis said something that helped me realize where my focus should be: "I don't know how to fix this or why this happened. But what I do know is that you have to get Kate well from this surgery, and then get her out of this hospital and home. Right now you have to concentrate on that and only that, and you have to do it one day at a time." I grabbed onto this thought like a lifeline.

My folks showed up next. "Please tell them not to come in," Kate said through her pain. "I know they care but if they come in I'll know what they're thinking and it will only make me sad and then it will take me hours to be happy again." And so I took my folks to the cafeteria as well. Diners coming in for lunch left us plenty of space as we hugged and wept. Mom squeezed me like she'd never let me go; Dad's lip quivered as he held my hand and quietly cried.

We were all overwrought. In a stressful moment, Ellen snapped aggressively at our doctor right in front of Kate. Kate pleaded with her not to interfere. Giff implored, "Ellen, come on!" Kate's sister Kim, a flight attendant who flew in shortly after the surgery, looked ashen. Ellen explained that in Kim's nursing days, she had cared for cancer patients, thus she knew what to expect.

"I used to work on the surgical floor with a lot of cancer patients," Kim has since told me. "I was thinking, 'Oh God, Kate has to go through all of that. The tube feedings and losing all the weight. It's horrible.' I remember looking at Kate, thinking she looks really healthy, and thinking that the next time I see her she's not going to look like that anymore. I wanted to stay and help her in any way I could.

"It didn't seem real to me," Kim continued. "I thought, 'Kate can't die, because she's too healthy. How come it happened to her and not me? It should have happened to me.' And I also just kept thinking, 'I can't live without my sister. This can't happen to our family. How come it's happening to our family? It's not fair.'" When Kim left to go back home to her husband, Dan, and her daughter—our niece—Laura, she was torn. "I don't want to leave you," she sobbed to Kate.

Amid all this turmoil and tears, I might have been the most useless of anyone. It was all I could do to keep a solid face in Kate's room before bursting into tears in the arms of loved ones in the hall.

And though much of the drama took place outside the room, Kate sensed it. Soon she told me that it was all going to bring her down. "I don't want to be part of somebody's tragedy," she said. "I don't want this to be some big emotional thing. I can't take it. I just want to be myself."

In the days following that third surgery I called a number of our friends to fill them in on the news. Those were difficult calls, but they strengthened Kate and me. Friends counseled me and I passed their messages on to Kate. One old friend said he would pray for us, even though I suspected he had never prayed in his life. Another friend suggested we start journals. Others said they would fly across the country in a minute if we needed them. Another offered to do whatever we wanted—act like everything was normal if that's what we needed. A bouquet of flowers arrived with a card that stated simply, "From your Bellingham family." Another friend said, "Give Kate two hugs from us and then have her give *you* one back from us." Still another friend, whose mother had died from cancer, said prophetically, "I'm so sorry for you, you have so much still to go through." A friend reported that his brother and sister-in-law had had a baby in Portland Thursday, shortly after we found out about Kate's recurrent cancer—life and death spiraled each other in an unending game.

Our friend Ellen Schmidt arrived at the room the day after the surgery, not knowing of Kate's results and prognosis. Kate's parents quickly ushered Ellen out of the room. I walked with her down the hall, explaining the results and how Kate didn't want to see anyone just then. Ellen helped me with my anguish. "Keep your faith," she said. "You two will work this out together just like everything else. Scott, remember, you cannot let her die here and now."

In the days ahead, Kate slowly moved through the stages of getting well from abdominal surgery—the breathing, the walking, the long wait for her bowels to start working again. One day when we were alone, I unabashedly passed gas. Kate gave me a sour look, then commented wryly, "Sure, that's easy for you to say."

"There's no rush for your bowels to start working," I told her. "The food in the cafeteria is awful. If you ate it, you would just die." I tried to grab the words and stuff them back in my mouth, but I couldn't. Kate ignored me.

The nurses somehow learned that Kate had been slated to run the Victoria Marathon. At separate times, two different nurses asked, "Weren't you supposed to run a marathon this week?" Both times Kate just shrugged, but she deflated like a balloon that had just been pricked. For her, every interaction was an exercise in mental gymnastics that had to be held and felt and judged against the pain it might cause.

One night in the hospital, Kate moaned, "Owee, Owee!" from the excruciating pain of a brutal headache. I raced for the nurse, who gave Kate a Tylenol. I cried silently, utterly hopeless as Kate agonized because all I could think of was *brain tumor* and how maybe she would die that night, and how maybe that would be good if that was the least painful thing for her, and how we were not ready yet, and how confused I was. How could it be, I thought, that just two weeks ago we were kayaking down the Stikine?

In another day or three, Kate passed a bit of gas, meaning that she could finally sip on some juice. I wept as I returned to the room after hearing this news from a nurse, unsure if my tears resulted from happiness at Kate's progress or sadness at the smallness of her achievement. My emotions were utterly muddled. Kate felt equally confused. "I kept going back and forth about what I'd do when they let me out of the hospital," Kate recalls. "More treatment? Go back to work?"

One thought cropped up in my mind over and over as the days went by: Even then, under a death sentence, Kate had only really been sick from cancer treatment, never from cancer. "Day by day I was recovering even faster than after the radical hysterectomy," Kate remembers. "I didn't feel all that bad." It was a realization that provided little comfort. Life's vibrancy centers on the expectations we hold for it. Suddenly we saw no future. "I had no idea what my next goal should be," she concludes.

Kate's catheter was removed. Then the leg squeezers came off. For the briefest moment I worried that Kate's leg swelling would return and thought about how sad it would make her, and then I realized how insignificant that problem now seemed. Slowly we moved toward being ready to go home—but for what? To die?

◪

Summer started the day Kate and I hiked around Black and Nevada Mountains. The temperature had climbed from the high 30s in recent days into the 80s. This being Montana, however, at day's end we found ourselves setting up the tent in a pounding hailstorm. After the hail passed, a late, orange sun showed low under the trailing edge of the thundercloud. The sun's cold rays illuminated the endless fields of larkspur surrounding our tent, throwing a soft purple glow over the meadow.

Shortly after we started the following morning, June 22, just before Stemple Pass, we saw another couple with backpacks approaching rapidly. The woman, slim and blonde, wore black tights. The man wore sunglasses and long underwear. He sported a scruffy face. Each wore running shoes and carried two ski poles. The poles flashed in the early morning sunlight as the couple glided down the road like a couple of cross-country skiers. Only the snow was missing.

We hailed them to stop and talk. "Wow, more hikers, our first since Glacier," we exclaimed.

"Us, too," they replied. Dan and Sara Rufner were from San Diego and had walked the Pacific Crest Trail (PCT) two years earlier. Like us they carried identical backpacks, ours from Dana Designs, theirs from Gregory.

I asked what it was like to hike in running shoes. Dan reported that they'd made the change on the PCT. "Too hot in the Mojave Desert to wear hiking boots," Dan explained.

"Did the Gear Nazi get to you?" I asked. They both laughed, knowing immediately that I referred to Ray Jardine, renowned in hiking circles both famously and infamously for his theories about lightweight, long-distance backpacking. It was Jardine who brilliantly wrote in his book *The Pacific Crest Trail Hiker's Handbook*, "If I need it and don't have it, I don't need it."

Dan, who did most of the talking, explained that they were hiking from Canada to Mexico along the CDT. "We're shooting for 23 miles a day."

Kate and I gulped. We mentioned that we hoped to make something like 10 or 11 miles a day, and that so far we had rarely achieved our goal.

Dan and Sara had come through Glacier Park, crossing some of the big snowfields that Kate and I had worried over, getting turned back once by the big storm that had changed our starting point from Waterton to the Belly River trailhead. Dan expressed some dismay that others he had heard of on the trail were not walking the entire CDT in a one-way path, like themselves, but instead jumping from New Mexico to Montana and so on to better work with the weather. A couple of times Dan asked if we planned to take the "Anaconda Cutoff," a fair diversion from the Divide's official trail, but a distinct favorite of most CDT hikers. Kate and I hadn't even heard of the Anaconda Cutoff. Dan and Sara recommended that we stay away from the rough Elk Mountain trail at the north end of the Bob Marshall Wilderness, "unless you're keen on taking the 'official' route." Dan and Sara, quite clearly, were keen on taking the official route.

While we talked, Dan and Sara fidgeted like two racehorses dying to get back to the track. Indeed, Dan had said earlier, "We're always working against time." On this day, they planned to cover the same distance Kate and I had walked in the past two days. As we parted, I asked them for an address so that we might contact them at the end of the summer. Sara handed me a business card that gave their website plus descriptions of two Christian charities they were earning funds for through people sponsoring their hike. Then off they went, ski poles flashing.

Walking on toward Stemple Pass, I considered our discussions with Dan and Sara. Long-distance hiking provides plenty of time for such rumination. Dan and Sara's goal, from what we had gathered, was to hike the entire 3,100-mile CDT in a single year, north to south, on the official trail. I began for the first time to seriously consider what had motivated Kate and me to undertake this hike. I soon came up with three simple reasons: first as a celebration of being alive, second because of our desire to explore Montana, and finally because of the physical challenge. Strangely, *completing* the Montana section of the CDT didn't even make the top three. Okay, to be fair, it was probably fourth.

Clearly goals are important. Goals drive greatness. Still, sometimes the goal can overshadow the value of the process. In this journey, as in our journey with cancer, Kate and I needed the path to be as important as the endpoint.

Leaving Dan and Sara, we headed two miles down the dirt road to Stemple Pass rather than hiking along the short section of trail they had just popped out from. And so here, as on the Belly River, as below Greenhorn Mountain, we were not on the "official" route. A part of me suspected that Dan and Sara were looking back and wondering why those silly hikers were taking the road rather than the trail. And another part of me wanted to yell, "We could do the whole thing, too—Canada to Mexico! And we could stay on the official route. And before cancer, maybe we would have. But we have lived through cancer and chemo and radiation and too many surgeries and we are so, so glad just to be here!"

Of course I didn't yell, and I felt immediately sheepish for even having the thought. But as Kate and I walked along the dirt road, a hundred yards off the official trail, I found it somewhat liberating to realize that I just didn't care. And later, sitting in the sun at Stemple Pass, I had an epiphany of sorts. I realized I like stopping to take pictures of flowers, and how Kate and I took time to read aloud to each other or make sushi at an extended lunch as we were doing just then. Perhaps I am getting less young, I thought.

I raised a silent water bottle toast to Dan and Sara. I applaud your vitality and marathoner looks and approach to the CDT. I probably envy your youth and definitely envy what I perceive to be your innocence. Kate and I no longer retain the luxury of innocence. When you reach the Mexican border, which I am almost certain you will, my new friends, I hope that you will pause long enough to realize the enormity of your accomplishment.

◪

It wasn't far into the day following the surgery, while I read to her, that Kate told me I needed to shave and look good if I planned to be her assistant in getting out of the hospital. "You've got to take care of yourself," she said in a strange transposition of roles. She knew that given my anxieties, I had not eaten at all during the days surrounding the surgery. "Eat something!" Kate admonished me through her pain. "You have to be strong if you're going to help me get out of here." I told her it wasn't fair that I could eat while she could not. Kate said not to worry, that it was American Dream pizza and Full Sail Ale in her IV.

Thus one night while Ellen sat with Kate, Giff, Kim, and I went to dinner. Giff said that we must—we *would*—somehow pull off a miracle cure for Kate. He had read that St. Augustine once said something to the effect that miracles are not aberrations of nature, but rather phenomena of nature we simply don't understand. Then the three of us talked about the idea of miracles and how they really do happen.

Yet I felt certain that if there really were a chance Kate might not be alive by the next summer, as the doctor had suggested, she would not want to spend her remaining days chasing around the world after cures. Many times in the past we had talked about what we'd do if Kate's death from cancer became imminent. "In the year we spent traveling in New Zealand," she had once said, "we lived a lifetime. So why would I chase after false hopes instead of enjoying the time I had left?"

Another night later in the week I went to dinner with Suz and Dennis, who stopped on their return from the Victoria Marathon. Hearing them talk about the race felt surreal, from a hazy place and time that we used to be a part of, a happy place that Kate and I could no longer touch. It was such a short time ago that we, too, had been training to run that marathon.

I returned to the room from dinner to find Kate crying frantically. Ellen said, "She needs you," and everyone quickly disappeared. Our doctor and his oncology nurse had just departed. Other than checking regularly on her healing progress, the doctor had not previously spoken directly to Kate about the surgical results. He presumed, I imagine, that her parents and I had done so. While we had told Kate about the remaining cancer, we had not told her of her doctor's prognosis.

Now that several days had gone by since the surgery and Kate had grown stronger, our doctor must have felt the appropriate time had come. What an incredibly tough job that must be, I realize now in retrospect, to present such horrible news to another person, all the while with emotional family hanging next to the bed. He started by giving Kate a photo of the remaining tumor. He told her that it would be difficult to treat it further. He then made a few comments about chemotherapy and radiation, but seemed understandably more comfortable slipping back into discussions of Kate's recovery from the trauma of surgery.

As the doctor moved to leave, Ellen implored, "You can't discharge her from the hospital without giving her some kind of a prognosis." Pushed to do so, the doctor told Kate that it didn't look good, that she had a one in ten chance of being alive for two years. All this, which had occurred just before I arrived, had resulted in Kate's hysterics and crying frenzy.

Tossing my coat aside, I tried to hold Kate but she convulsed and twisted so violently that I could not, and I worried she might rip out her IV. She wept uncontrollably. Her eyes quickly puffed up and when I tried to look into them my heart broke in two. It felt like death had arrived in our room. Kate finally let me hold her, her writhing slowing, and she began to sob into my shoulder. I quieted her and tried to say the right things, but I could think of no right things. After some time Kate started to breathe more slowly. Giff and Ellen came back into the room and we all held Kate at once.

Later, while Kate was in the bathroom, I told Giff, "I'm no good at this. I don't have any practice."

Giff replied quietly, "None of us do."

◪

Kate and I continued north from Stemple Pass through beautiful forest with lush undergrowth. For a great distance the trail contoured a steep hill slope, dazzling in its carpet of green. Three mountain bikers—the only three we would see on CDT single track the entire summer—kindly yielded the trail. They were riding from Flesher Pass to Stemple Pass, then on into Lincoln. What a contrast the mountain bikers provided to the four loud OHV riders that raced past us on a previous day. The bikers approached silently, and we noticed their approach only when they rounded a corner directly ahead.

Pushing toward Flesher Pass, Kate walked with joy and bounce for a second day straight. I felt ecstatic. Our renewed strength signaled that we were up to the demands of the trail. Plus, with over a hundred miles under our belts, I reckoned we had at least moved out of the weekend backpacker's realm. Still, I wondered, "How will we hold up during the second hundred miles, the third, and the fourth?"

As if in answer, nine or ten miles into the day Kate fell to the ground like a sack of potatoes. I ran to her because the fall looked so bizarre. There had been no root to trip her up; she simply collapsed in a heap. By the time I reached her, Kate was already rising. Though I asked several times, she would give no explanation, nothing about being faint or her knees suddenly buckling. She said, "I'm fine. Stop worrying. Let's go and find a place to camp." Still, as we walked on I was forced to wonder, Are we too close to some edge? Are we pushing too hard?

Beyond Flesher Pass, we climbed though forest and lupine meadows to a ridge top for lunch. A cool breeze chilled us. Thunderclouds piled up far back to the west. Dark, heavy clouds hovered ominously ahead while pillowy clouds lazed their way into the valleys below. As we climbed on, those clouds pushed up from the valleys. Soon mist enveloped us and we could not see 30 yards ahead.

For four hours we walked in the clouds. This must be how an angel feels, I thought. The track at times grew scant, and we labored to find trail markings and turns. If Kate got 50 yards ahead, I had to yell to find her. The clouds held cool mist, but the air stood eerily calm. We hiked across ridges and over saddles, through meadows and down lonely logging roads, all the while trapped inside a moving 30-yard half sphere. In burned areas, tree skeletons became ghosts at the edge of our bubble, then mysteriously disappeared.

Tiring, we stopped in a small grove of trees and set up the tent. I dropped down the hill and found a spring for water. As I walked back, a fresh breeze rustled the treetops. Thunder sounded off to the west, though our soft half sphere of clouds hid us from the world. We made hot cocoa over an open fire, then started pasta. It began to drizzle. More distant thunder sounded and then came a visible lightning flash, close at hand. The rain strengthened and the wind began to push hard. We piled wood on the fire and fled for the tent as the storm ratcheted into a tempest. The thunder moved closer. Rain pounded the tent. More and more lightning flashed, each time illuminating the inside of our shelter for an eerie moment.

"Let's lie on the foam pads," Kate urged, "they'll insulate us from the ground." An electrical engineer is a good partner to have in a lightning storm.

I looked at my watch to count the seconds between lightning flashes and booms of thunder. Twenty seconds, twelve, nine, seven. At five seconds, Kate grabbed my hand. "If we're going to fry, let's fry together." We smiled weakly at each other, understanding that she had not meant to be funny.

Then three seconds, two, and finally one and a half seconds between the thunder and lightning. We were 500 meters horizontally from the bolt with no vertical buffer. With each flash we cringed. We weren't *in* the storm; we *were* the storm. For 75 minutes rain and thunder and lightning sounded in concert. The thunder and lightning counts stayed under five seconds for what seemed like an eternity. With every thunder boom I understood the analogy between thunder and the gods bowling—we had camped on the headpin.

Slowly the booms moved to 8 seconds apart, then 14 seconds, 26 seconds, and finally a minute apart. The thunder that had started on the Lincoln side of the tent now sounded from the Helena side. The pounding rain now pattered. We climbed out of the tent into a light mist. The clouds had lifted and our small bubble of limited visibility had disappeared. We found ourselves camped directly on the spine of the continent. As if embarrassed by its absence, the sun slipped its last rays of the day under the trailing clouds. Toward Helena the heavy thunderheads continued their onslaught of the eastern face of the Rockies. Lightning bolts rocketed downward. To the south, the trail we had hiked in the clouds climbed up a ridge and across the mountaintops. Its wet surface shone like a golden thread in the cold sunshine.

Back at the campfire, we found no flame, no hot coals even. But we did find pleasingly cooked, still-warm noodles.

◪

The second day after we learned of Kate's cancer recurrence, I began a daily run. At first I balked at Kate's suggestion that I go, telling her I didn't think it was fair for me to go running when she couldn't. Moments earlier she had taken her first struggling steps away from the bed. She lay back down, exhausted by her effort. "I just finished my run for the day—now go!" she urged me with half-closed eyes. "You'll feel better. Run for both of us."

After that I ran every day on the peaceful trails of Forest Park and on those closer to the hospital. The runs cleared out the stuffiness of the hospital from my head but in turn made room for horrible thoughts. My mind swung wildly. I worried about the day's trials and then projected myself into a frightening future.

One day all I could think about was Kate dying, and what I would say at a memorial service. I pictured a large group of people, an invitation telling no one to wear black or formal clothes, that while this was a sad moment about death, it was also a moment for celebrating life. I thought of the things I wanted to tell them about Kate, and I knew that I would not be able to get through them all. I would say that this is a time for us all to open our hearts to nothing else but Kate, a time to remember how she touched each one of us in whatever special way.

The gathering in my mind occurs at night because I want to show slides of Kate. I tell them that while cancer was what defined Kate's last moments on earth, Kate was not about cancer. "That's why so few of you saw her for the last few weeks," I say, "because that sickly body was not Kate and she did not want you to think of her that way. Instead she would want us to remember her as a person who loved life. She was a private person who valued friendship and quiet times and rational thought and running and health."

As I headed down through the forest, a drizzle began. I rounded a corner, 35 minutes into the run, and tried to hide my tears from a young couple hiking toward me. Once I was past them, I started projecting again. I thought of myself at 60, downtrodden, cursing the life I'd had to live without Kate. I thought of things that I would promise her before she died: that I would think of her every day and that every time I looked at Orion's belt—a constellation she first showed me—I would think of her and hope she was thinking of me. I thought of how hard it would be to explain to someone else that though I might be with them, I could never love again as completely as I loved Kate. I wondered if anyone would have me, knowing this.

And then I thought that Kate and I would promise each other things. I thought that I would *re*marry her before she died. And I thought that I would ski her ashes up the tiny valley we love in Montana and pour the ashes into the stream so that they could be distributed by the clear waters.

Much of the time I cried as I ran, and I thought that if Kate knew she would tell me how pitiful I was. All the while I cried because her footsteps weren't echoing right behind me, and I wasn't sure if they ever would be again.

◪

We hit the trail at 7 A.M., hoping to quickly hike to Rogers Pass, then hitchhike to Lincoln in time for the Fourth of July parade. The cold morning and remnants of moisture from the previous night's storm left the valleys below us blanketed under cotton ball clouds. The clouds covered Lincoln and everything else north and west of us right up to 6,000 feet. We stood in delicious morning sunshine and felt like we were atop Denali or maybe Everest. To the west and north, only the peaks of the Scapegoat and Bob Marshall Wilderness areas reached into the sunshine. To the east, out across the Rocky Mountain Front, the clouds spilled out onto the flat plate of the plains and quickly dissipated. The Little Belts and the Big Belts stood tall in the sun, throwing shadows westward. Closer at hand, two tawny deer emerged from the clouds below us and climbed into the morning light. Kate and I stood there on the top of the world, awestruck by it all, feeling as if the hand of God was reaching down and touching us. At that moment, more than any since the journey had started, we knew that the hike was right.

For three hours we walked our ridge of sun, our packs light, the distance short, and our minds fully aware. The clouds hung heavy enough that they had not dissipated by the time we reached the high ridge that looks down into Rogers Pass. At the pass, a woman from Great Falls, Colleen, drove us 18 miles down into the fog to Lincoln. She had watched the lightning display the previous night for hours and felt confident that it would prove more exciting than the Missoula fireworks she planned to see that night. Colleen told us that the storm had brought a freakish tornado that tore the roof off a trailer home near Great Falls. It had also dumped an inch of rain in 20 minutes in Missoula and left behind golf-ball-sized hail.

At 10 A.M., Colleen dropped Kate and me at Lambkins, her favorite Lincoln breakfast spot. The place was jammed when we walked in, then emptied as though someone had yelled "Fire!" Kate and I huddled inconspicuously into a corner booth, hoping to hide our odoriferous offenses, but the waitress assured us that the other customers had departed to get a good spot for the Fourth of July parade. We ate alone, heartily, and then found a place among the folks lining Main Street.

Parades in small western towns run predictably and this one did not disappoint. Small town parades start with floats, *real* floats built on flatbeds and pulled by Ford F350s. The first is sponsored by the local hardware store and carries a square dancing group a whoopin' and a hollerin'. Then comes a float with country and western singers, then one with the rodeo queen and her court. Next come the horsemen and women: a sheriff's posse, the local Forest Service folks, an outfitter leading his band of loaded mules, some rodeo riders, and then a cowboy lassoing a gal running around in a clown suit complete with flaming red hair and floppy shoes.

Next come the automobiles. Many are polished classic cars that have been driven across the state just for the parade. Others are hot rods—some are new, some are rusted. Then starts a grand small town parade tradition, the great revving of the internal combustion engine. Every roar of the V-8 brings hoots from the crowd. If the proud hot rod owner can squeal his tires (sorry, ladies, these are almost inevitably men) without running over the unlucky entrant in front of him, well, all the better. Somewhere along the way comes a giant convertible, carrying the mayor or parade master or whoever else can look sufficiently official in a Stetson, bolo tie, and corduroy sport jacket. The convertible—a car no one in the six surrounding counties would ever consider buying—comes from a local car dealership, with signs on all four sides announcing that fact. Near the end of the car lineup someone slips in with a dilapidated '74 Datsun, "Hey, dude, this ain't Macy's," he yells out the window. "I just want to be in a parade!"

Arms flash out from every car window to sprinkle candy on the ground. Kids scatter to retrieve the pieces while moms yell, "Don't step in those horse apples!" Adults hand over the small hard candies to their kids while stealthily slipping the chocolates into their own pockets.

Now come the walkers and the late entrants. The clown has returned. A go-cart loops through the crowd, closely pursued by an OHV, both driven by teenage boys. A small girl, her mother discreetly following, pulls a wagon loaded with puppies. Someone on a unicycle shoots water into the crowd and proves himself less than popular. Next come a string of miniature ponies, then a woman leading a llama, and then three teenage boys in patched bell-bottoms that drag on the ground.

And finally, in small town parade tradition, comes the grand finale— the noisemakers. First the sheriff, lights flashing, hits his siren. The volunteer fire department, new truck shining, adds its call to the hullabaloo. In a moment the driver of a semi truck, reacting to the arm motions of the kids, pulls on his air horn. A local tow truck just behind lets loose. The din quickly grows unbearable; mothers grab for their children's ears, yet still everyone smiles.

And then, being that the town and the parade are short, they do it all over again.

As with all small town parades, there was a singular constant throughout that Fourth of July parade in Lincoln. Everyone, whether in the crowd or a parade participant, waved. They switched arms when the first arm tired and then waved some more until it seemed like the parade was some alien plot to have everyone recognize their neighbors for once and smile. And maybe that is exactly what a parade should be about.

The parade over, Kate and I moved to Leeper's Motel, where owners Bob and Margaret proceeded to make us feel at home. Though they had no rooms available, they allowed us to use the hot tub and to camp under an enormous ponderosa pine behind the motel. Once we had our tent up, we walked around town, stopping at Garland's for supplies and then the Lincoln Lodge for dinner. Back at Leeper's much later, Margaret lamented that Kate and I had spent hours walking even though we were supposed to be having a half day off.

"Tonight it'll be another two miles up to the park to see the fireworks," she said. "You two shouldn't be walking on your rest day. You can just drive our truck up."

We thanked Margaret for her kind offer but in the end never made use of the truck. Both Kate and I fell asleep before dark. When the first boom announced the 10:30 start of the fireworks, I rolled over, unzipped the tent door, and considered walking out to the highway to get a view past the monstrous ponderosa grove where we had camped. A moment later I dropped my head to the pillow, content with seeing three whitetail deer grazing just in front of the tent.

◣

For those of us pacing the hospital halls that week after the cancer-rediscovering surgery, faith and positive thought provided our only respite. "Don't lose your faith in God," Elaine, the patient Kate had started out sharing a room with, told me. She lay in her bed with IV lines connected, her face lined and wan. I stood in the doorway of her room. "God can make Kate well and take care of you both. All you have to do is ask."

"Kate and I are best friends," I said to Elaine, trying to steer the conversation away from a discussion of religion. "Our psyches are so intertwined that sometimes we seem like one person, thinking, feeling, even saying the same things at the exact same moment."

"Jesus is the best friend anyone can ever have," she said, steering the conversation back where she wanted it. "The earth is the closest to heaven you'll get without Jesus and the closest to hell you'll get with Jesus." So I told her that I just kept trying, but maybe I didn't get it. I prayed hard and tried to make contact, but I did not always know if anyone was listening.

Kate's mom Ellen told us about a friend of a friend who was still alive six years after cancer treatments, even though the doctors had given her just six months to live. "The spirit can do amazing things," Ellen said from the heart. I asked if the woman had adenocarcinoma like Kate. "I didn't ask," Ellen replied. "I just wanted to focus on the positives."

Ellen and Giff are solid Catholics. On the day our doctor had told Kate of her prognosis, when Kate collapsed in tears, Giff had come to her and said, "It's going to be okay. Fifty-four days ago I started a novena for you, before we even knew you were sick again. I finished the novena today. In the past I've seen a sign at the end of the novena, four roses. Today your mother and I drove into a park and we stopped, my mind blank. Then I looked up and right in front of us we saw a tall bush with roses in bloom, four splendid red roses. I told your mother about the sign and it was like a huge weight had been removed from my body."

Giff remembers thinking that those of us listening to him must have thought he'd fallen off the deep end. But he felt joy in being able to relate his sign to Kate and in seeing her eyes wanting to believe him. "I knew she would be okay," he said later, "if she could only believe."

Through all the family and friends, crying and pain, Kate's recovery from her third surgery progressed. She soon stood uncertainly beside the bed, and then sat in a chair. We made a game out of her breath-measuring device, and always she tried to pull more and more air into her lungs. On the second night after surgery, Kate woke at 4 A.M. and told me she wanted to get up and stretch. Half asleep, I rolled over and said something intelligent like, "Huh? What?"

Kate's determined stare pierced the darkened room. "Are you sure?" I said, coming awake. "What about your stitches?" Kate *demanded* that we get up. We struggled to get her standing, struggled to keep the tubes and catheters from tangling in her movements. For ten minutes she did arm twirls and leg bends, grimacing through the pain of the stitches in her abdomen. When she lay down, I massaged her legs.

As soon as Kate could stand, she wanted to walk—first to the door, then down the halls of 5C. Soon the walks got longer: out to the sky bridge, then across the sky bridge to the VA hospital, then across the sky bridge and around the VA. We walked often, sometimes as much as a mile. Those walks were important. Every walk brought Kate renewed color and vigor.

Several mornings after the surgery, as sunlight streamed through the window, our doctor came in with his residents and a group of medical students. While they discussed Kate's recovery from surgery, the doctor lifted the bandage off Kate's scar. "We broke a needle on your stomach muscles," one of the residents told Kate.

As the doctor and his entourage left, Kate whispered to me, "Muscles of woven steel."

One night, pausing on the sky bridge after our longest walk yet, we watched the lights of the city. People in cars below were moving unperturbed about their daily lives. Later, pushing the IV pole ahead, we returned to the room but did not turn on the lights. I cracked the window because even though it was October, the room felt hot and musty. Kate did not want to get back into bed, so instead we rearranged the catheters and tubing, then stood between the bed and the window and held each other.

Slowly, gently, an eerie yet delightful sound floated in from outside. Five stories below a lone man sat on a concrete loading dock playing quiet blues on a harmonica. As the man swayed back and forth, his soulful tune echoed off the concrete walls behind him. Standing silently, Kate and I held each other in the darkness, listening. I sensed that some of our fears seemed to dissipate just then because that special moment, like the walks, belonged to Kate and me, no one else. Cancer could not take it from us.

◤

On the morning we planned to head back onto the trail, the postmaster searched in vain for our supply package at the Lincoln post office. Friendly chaos filled the place. Our package was nowhere to be found among the disjointed stacks of mail. Yet we felt confident in our package's existence. Two Corvallis friends, Doug and Darcy, had been studiously sending our packages along the way, often adorning the boxes with photos, poetry, and wise maxims. After three searches through the stacks, the postmaster consented to let Kate join the search back in the mailroom and soon our package magically materialized. Just try getting behind the counter and sorting your own mail in Los Angeles—or even Bozeman!—we thought.

Sitting on the loading dock behind the post office, I opened an unremarkable envelope. A newspaper clipping fell out. Bold, black letters on the headline read "Tijeras Woman Loses Life in Collision on Old Hwy 66." Below the headlines was a photo of Harriet Goodness. My mouth dropped and I went limp, surrendering the letter to Kate. She read the obituary aloud and soon our eyes welled with tears.

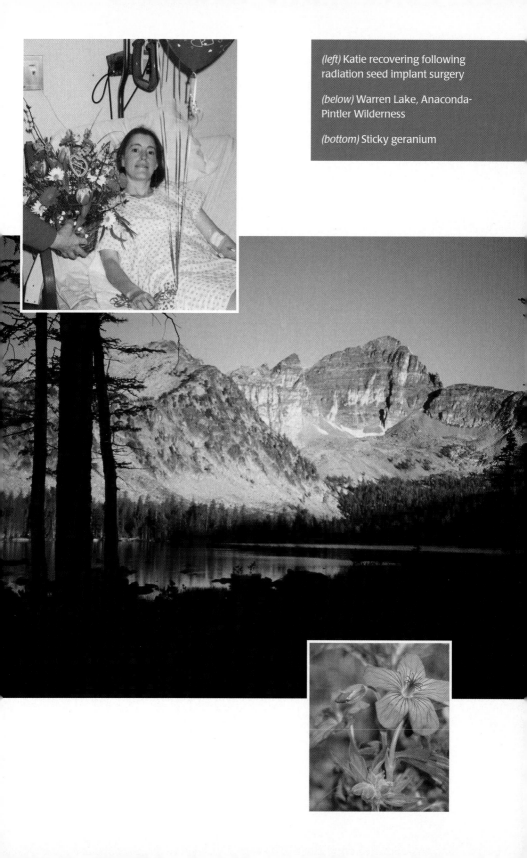

(left) Katie recovering following radiation seed implant surgery

(below) Warren Lake, Anaconda-Pintler Wilderness

(bottom) Sticky geranium

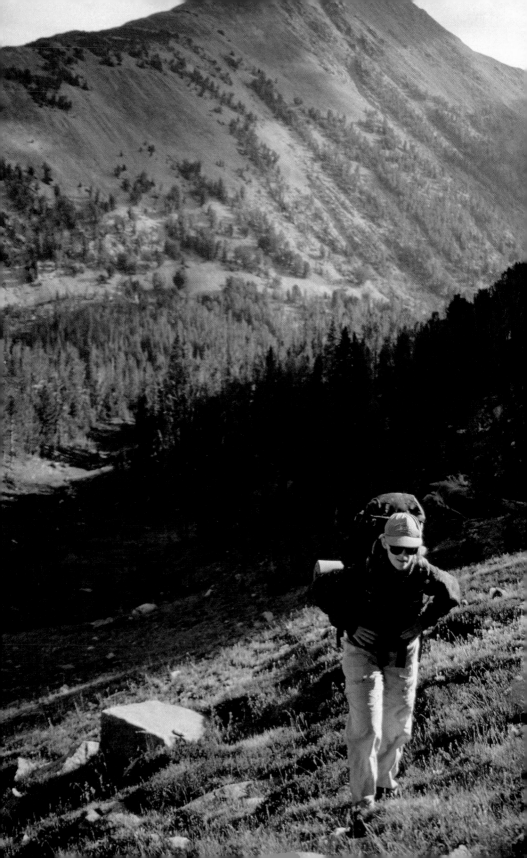

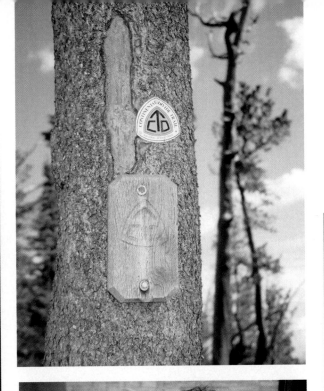

(opposite) Near Squaw Mountain, in the Bitterroot Range

(top) Tree blaze, plus old and new CDT reassurance symbols

(bottom) Preparing food for three months on the trail

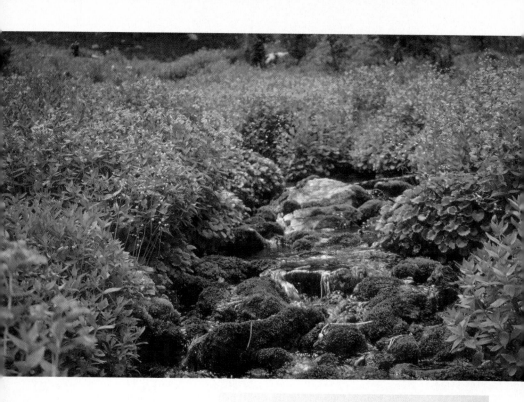

(above) Monkey flowers

(right) Katie with Ranger Bob in Glacier National Park

(opposite) Bighorn ram near Piegan Pass, Glacier National Park

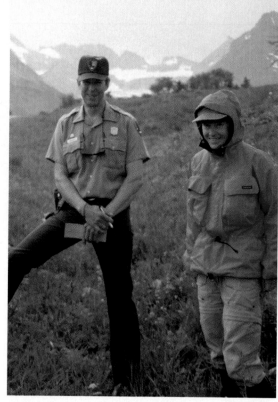

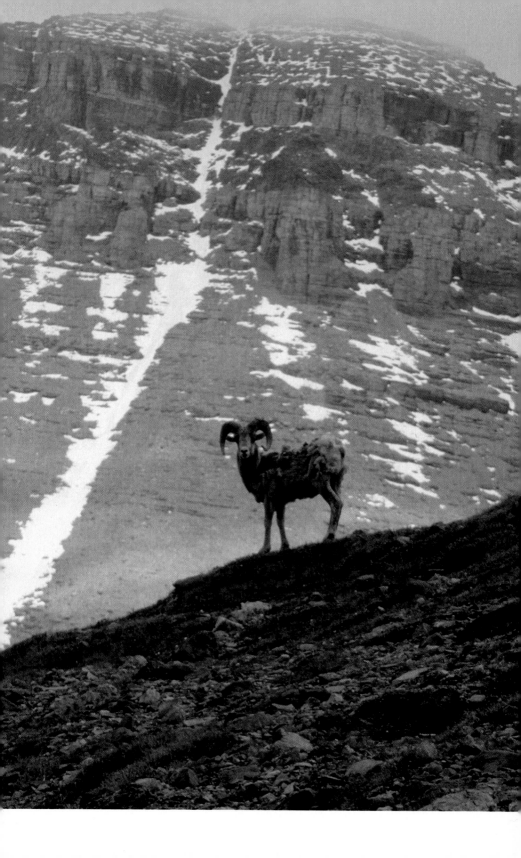

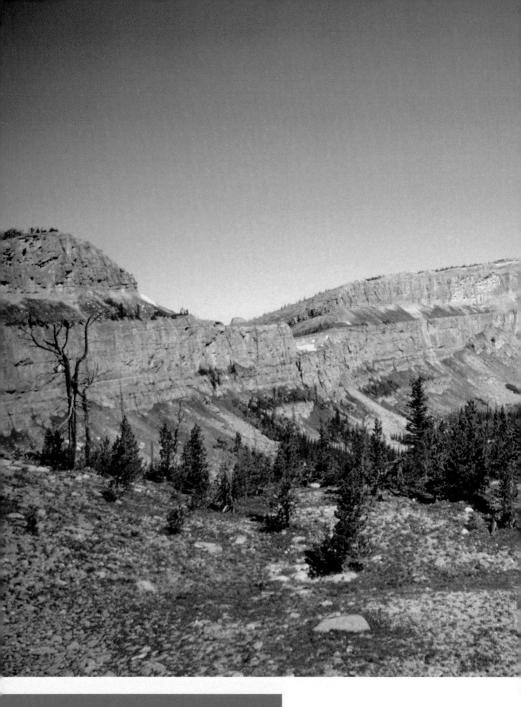

(above) The Chinese Wall, Bob Marshall Wilderness

(opposite, top) Katie and Tigger, resting at home

(opposite, bottom) On a short walk while waiting for surgery number four

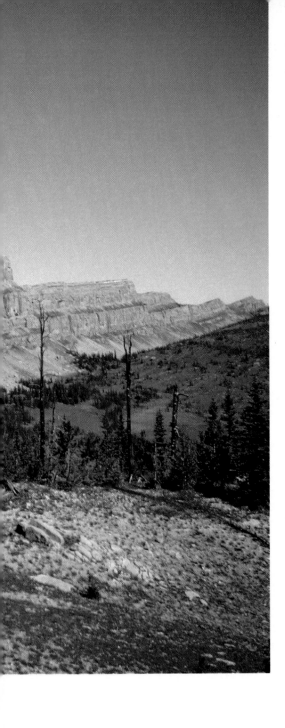
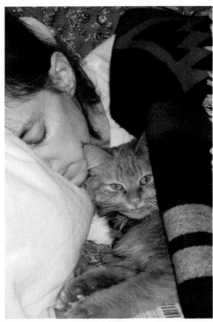
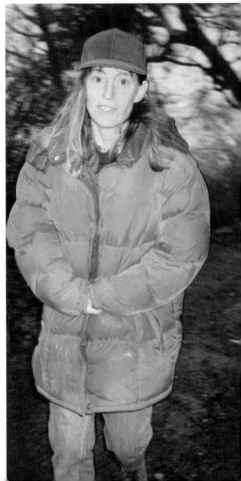

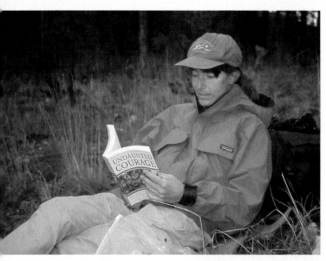

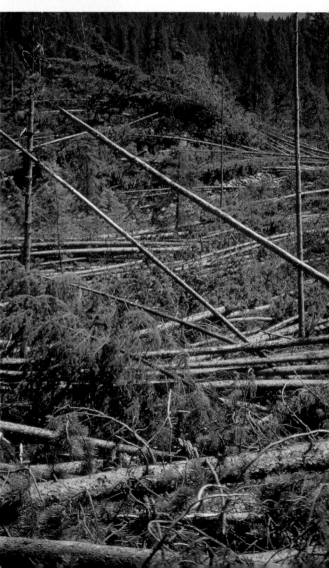

(top) Katie reading near Schultz Saddle, Beaverhead-Deerlodge National Forest

(right) Thunderbolt Creek blowdown

Harriet was a woman from whom I rented a room in the early '80s while I worked as a postgraduate intern at Albuquerque's Sandia National Laboratories. Silver-haired, sun-hardened, and slim, Harriet had a ready laugh and the vibrancy and zeal of a teenager. She wrote to us once about going to her 45th high school reunion and joked about seeing "all those old people!" She loved her dogs, her church, her cross-country skiing and whitewater rafting, her jug band, and her Budweiser. Harriet was a great housemate who became an even better friend in the years after I left New Mexico. In recent years, she had frequently written to inquire about Kate's cancer treatments.

A couple of years back, as Kate was returning to health, Harriet wrote to say that she herself had lung cancer. Surgery removed the cancer, but it returned in other locations in subsequent years. Harriet's letters, which I'll piece together here, show her animated, infectious spirit:

Scott & Katie –

RATS! I thought by now you'd be at a beach somewhere. I was sorry to hear that you had another surgery. Enough already. Hope you continue to heal and let's hope that's the end of it.

I just canceled my vacation. . . . Looks like I've lived long enough to start wearing out body parts. June 8th I go in for hip replacement surgery. OUCH. . . . Let's swap prayers, huh?

In preparation for hip surgery, they found a spot on my lung! Going into surgery tomorrow 16th for lung cancer surgery . . . Shit! Praying. Hope Katie's doing better.

Thanks for sharing your GOOD NEWS with me. . . . Hope you continue to do well, Katie—there's so many roads to travel, eh?

The retirement party was incredible . . . 115 people. A keg is usually a good draw!!! . . . I designed and built a brand new house. . . . Had an open house a couple weeks ago. I told everyone not to bring anything . . . if they insisted on bringing something, bring bird food and/or wildflower seeds. Well, I ended up with 6 new birdhouses, 200 lbs of bird food, and many tins of flower seeds!!

Have been battling cancer—again—since this past June. Stayed reasonably drunk for a week—then pulled myself together and got on with it. None of the chemo into the bladder seems to be doing anything. . . .

Have fired my oncologist—all she did was tell me that without surgery I was going to die in a short time. So be it. They ain't gonna start carving on me!! I finally got pissed off and told her I was going to Ireland. She informed me I didn't have that much time left! Oh YEAH? Screw you, lady, I said, as I left the office for the last time.

Found a new doc at the UNM Cancer Treatment Center—instant rapport. He said he's kept another ole girl alive for 15 years with the same thing I've got. So we set up a plan, I went to Ireland, and upon return started more treatments under his care. Last biopsy in early September showed no sign of cancer YAY YAY YAY YAY YAY. I whooped and hollered all the way home.

I am so happy for you both. You had an awful time for a while. I know what you mean—every day has new meaning and every day you praise the Lord that you're still here and happy. Life is good. I keep waking up everyday. Take good care of yourselves. Give each other a hug from me.

Love, Harriet

Harriet beat her cancer through a combination of medical intervention, outdoor living, the support of church friends and, above all, pure orneriness. Retired, cancer-free, and living in a new home in the mountains she loved, Harriet was killed in a freak auto accident when a runaway trailer careened into her car on a windy New Mexico road.

There are many ways to die; cancer is only one. May we live with half the verve of this marvelous woman.

There at the post office I wrote our short epitaph in the CDT log:

It is an honor, privilege, and joy to walk Montana's Continental Divide. A day off brings a chance to reconnect with friends and family. Our stay here in Lincoln was bittersweet, however, as we just learned of the death of a friend—Harriet Goodness—a lover of life and of things wild. We will walk forward today for her.

And so, dear Harriet, we will miss you, your hearty laugh, your wit, your zest. Both of us thought of you as we climbed away from Rogers Pass. At one point Kate sat down and cried loudly, agonizing, "It just isn't fair. How can this happen to such a good person?" Sitting there in the scree on the side of Green Mountain I had no acceptable answer, so I simply held her.

◤

Discharge day finally arrived. If you're eating well and walking long distances, they send you home. Studies show that recuperation at home, when medically feasible, is faster than in the hospital. That knowledge is of little comfort when you are heading home after being told you will soon die. Yes, we wanted Kate home, and the sooner the better. But with the prognosis so dire, it felt more like she was being kicked out than released, like they needed the bed and no longer felt any responsibility for her well-being.

Our frustration was already high because of the talks we'd had with our doctor's chief oncology nurse in the days before Kate was discharged. The nurse had found an open Taxol treatment protocol for cervical cancer patients. Unfortunately, the nurse explained, the patient had to match certain criteria to be admitted to the study. Kate did not match those criteria. Kate and I are engineers, so the idea of a controlled study testing only certain parameters certainly did not come as a new concept. But we had already sat through discussions about pain management for terminal cancer patients, so you can't imagine our frustration at hearing the nurse say that Kate did not qualify for a new treatment protocol *that might save her life*. Later, stopping in to Kate's room, our doctor had helped minimize the frustration, saying he was willing to provide Kate the same treatment as the experimental protocol, though not as a part of the official study.

An hour before departing the hospital, Kate and I met with our doctor and his nurse together. They gave us their thoughts on potential follow-up treatments, mainly chemotherapy and radiation. Given that the side effects were ugly and that the odds of success low, our doctor suggested that one possible approach was to do nothing. His nurse spoke with great sincerity about what we could expect—further treatment or not—

including dietary restrictions, energy loss, and pain. Her descriptions were so matter-of-fact that for a moment we could almost forget that every statement she made implied another step down in life quality, another step toward Kate's predicted death.

Our doctor also talked about taking Kate's case to the hospital tumor board, in hopes of getting further thoughts on treatment possibilities. Unfortunately, we would have to wait for the board's next meeting, later that month. How, we wondered, could we be presented with the imminence of death on one hand, and then sit and patiently wait for a group of unknown doctors to gather at their leisure to consider Kate's fate?! How could we be asked to live by the board's time frame with the ticktock of our own clock growing deafening?

And how, we agonized, can we go home and live, given the expectation that only death awaits?

FIVE

Long Days

It is not easy to remember that in the fading light of day . . .
the shadows always point toward the dawn.

WINSTON O. ABBOTT
as quoted in *Cry of the Kalahari* by Mark and Delia Owens

From Kate's journal:

October 11, 1994. We came home from the hospital today. The three
things I wanted to do were to pet Tigger, to call my brother because I
haven't talked to him yet, and to start a journal. When we pulled
into the driveway there were a whole bunch of pumpkins with black
magic-markered faces on them. First we said our neighbor's kids,
Logan and Drew, did them and then we thought Rob and Rachel did
them because they're like a couple of kids. Cam and Terri started the
idea by bringing over the first three and then everyone else brought
over pumpkins that were self-portraits. They said welcome home and
we love you. The one Randy and Kelly did was carved intricately and
looked like the moon or something.

We brought home seven sets of flowers and they look great
around the house. Our neighbors Scott and Susan left the mail for us
and left us six-week muffin mix in the fridge. We can bake them as
we want to eat them. Scott's parents left us homemade chicken
noodle soup and some bread.

Tigger was really happy and has gained a few pounds. She has to be wherever I am. She needs a bath so she doesn't look so fluffy.

It is great to be home and to have freedom to do whatever I want. It is so quiet. We really like the quiet.

I learned a lot after my surgery about what will happen to my life in the next few years. All the new information doesn't exactly say what will happen to me because still a whole range of things could happen. But the general thought is that my cancer will start affecting my body in a year or two or maybe longer and probably kill me. It will take about a month to rest up from surgery and in about three weeks I could start radiation therapy.

The radiation is supposed to kill the cancer cells and zap other good cells in organs. It'll make me puke and have diarrhea and have food intolerance and get a small bladder. Scott already has a small bladder so we'll be the same after that. Six weeks of radiation and a month of recovery and I'll feel fine but the cancer will spread and kill me. The dose that the body can tolerate probably won't be enough to kill all of the cancer.

I was told I have 12 to 23 months left.

◤

Shortly after leaving Leeper's Motel the morning of July 6, we met Nick Williams, another CDT hiker. Nick waved us down in the middle of the highway. He said he'd heard there were other long-distance hikers in town. "I was looking at people coming in and out of Lambkins this morning, but none of them had the legs for it. Glad we ran into each other." A car honked to move us. When he learned we planned to hitchhike back to Rogers Pass, Nick said we might be able to catch a ride up with two folks, Gordon and Sue, who were helping Nick on his bid to walk the entire 3,100 miles of the CDT.

It only took a moment for us to register that Gordon and Sue were *the* Gordon and Sue of Continental Divide walking fame. We'd seen them in a video about the CDT and read about them in the book *Where the Waters Divide*. Gordon and Sue are a brother and sister from Missouri. They hiked avidly until Sue developed diabetes and became legally blind. For a few summers, Gordon would later explain, they toured and traveled, but found the change from hiking less than satisfying.

"We tried just camping," Gordon told us, "but we needed a purpose, a goal."

Somewhere along the way Gordon and Sue hit on an intriguing idea: Why not help other long-distance hikers achieve their goals of walking the CDT, PCT, AT, or Great Northern Trail? That was 15 years ago, and they've been at it most every summer since. Each year Gordon and Sue hook up with a hiker—"our hiker," Gordon had said—and provide shuttle service, food drops, and friendship for the months ahead.

This year Gordon and Sue had been shepherding two hikers: Nick, whom we had just met, and Ed Talone. Gordon and Sue had been helping Ed along in New Mexico when they met up with Nick and took him on as well.

Nick and Ed were tackling the Divide in a manner best suited to the vagaries of weather and snow, following a plan formulated to maximize the hiker's odds of completing the entire CDT in a single season. The hiker starts walking north from the Mexican border in April, crossing New Mexico while the weather remains cool. Cold and snow at the high elevations in Colorado's San Juan Mountains mandate a jump to southern Wyoming in late May. By mid to late June, Wyoming's Wind River Range south of Yellowstone Park necessitates another jump, this time to just north of the high peaks in Montana's Anaconda–Pintler Wilderness. Pushing north from there, the hiker hits the Scapegoat, Bob Marshall, and Glacier high country after the worst of the snow has melted out. On reaching the Canadian border, the hiker flip-flops back to hike south from the Pintlers through southwest Montana, Yellowstone, and the Wind River Range. Then it's another hop down to the Wyoming–Colorado border, and the crunch is on to walk the high peaks of Colorado before the winter snows fly.

Nick and Ed sat plunk in the middle of just such a route when we met them. With so much hopping around, it's apparent why help from Gordon and Sue is regarded as heaven-sent! Unfortunately, Ed was on this day prematurely ending his hike of the CDT; an important family matter called.

"I guess that means *I'm* Gordon and Sue's hiker now," Nick told us.

Nick introduced us to Gordon and Sue at their motel. Sue was small and gaunt, with wrinkled skin and age spots. Because of diabetes, she had lost most of her eyesight, been on dialysis, and undergone two kidney transplants, the first kidney coming from Gordon. Though she could make out shapes, she generally walked with Buddy, her Seeing Eye dog. Even with these challenges, Sue exuded vigor. Gordon said that when they're assisting hikers, Sue often walks 10 to 15 miles per day. Sue and Buddy walk up the trail, leaving balloons along the way to let their hiker know that food and the shuttle are near at hand. Sue inspired us—a remarkable woman staring into the face of great adversities and simply saying, "I will continue to be me!"

Nick still needed another hour to get ready, so Gordon wedged our backpacks into the van for the ride to Rogers Pass. Sue decided to stay behind, but sent Buddy along with us because she didn't want any of Lincoln's free-ranging mongrels attacking him. She wrapped a white handkerchief around her walking stick and went off for a stroll around town.

Kate squeezed herself into the backseat while I sat in the front of the van with Gordon. Buddy sat on the floorboards between us. Gordon wore a well-loved T-shirt that revealed a slightly protruding stomach. His bespectacled face held a stubbly beard and kindness. The old van reflected the nomadic lifestyle Gordon and Sue live for much of the year. Gear flowed freely out of every corner. A rickety shelf, its bolts long loosened from the ceiling and floor, teetered behind the driver's seat. Food and medicine bottles and books littered the dashboard. Most impressively, Gordon had taped a beautiful *National Geographic* page—complete with alpine scenery and wildflower photos—to the driver's side of the windshield, partially blocking his view.

Kate asked Gordon how much hiking *he* was doing. Gordon chuckled and said, "These days I spend most of my time driving, eating, and getting fat." When I told him I felt I was meeting someone famous, at least in CDT circles, Gordon guffawed. "Sometimes we wonder why we do these things—you know, drive people around who are stupid enough to strap 50 pounds on their backs and climb steep mountains. Then we drive down the interstate and see who the *really* crazy people are!"

We thanked Gordon profusely at Rogers Pass. He bid us good hiking and said he wished we'd had more time together. We wished the same, but Gordon and Sue would be moving north with Nick much more rapidly than us. They planned to meet Nick with food in Benchmark in three and a half days. We wouldn't be there for seven.

Heading up away from Rogers Pass, we met a horseman heading south down to the road. Gerald Larsen of Polson, Montana, looked like a frontiersman stepping out of mid-1800s Montana. He wore faded Wranglers, leather chaps, a torn flannel shirt, and a weathered cowboy hat. The heels of his cowboy boots were deeply worn. Behind Gerald's horse followed a pack donkey loaded with bulging panniers and a cloth-wall tent. Gerald carried a holstered six-shooter.

Gerald was the only horseman we met who was specifically out to follow the CDT. Like us, he hoped to cross Montana. Gerald asked where to pick up the trail on the other side of Rogers Pass, and about campsites and water availability. We filled him in, then returned the questions for our northward journey.

"Mostly the trail's pretty straightforward, well-marked, easy to follow." Gerald's slow drawl did nothing to diminish his frontiersman image. "Didn't have much problem. Should be easier for you to find, too, since you're going up an' all."

Then, from his perch in the saddle, Gerald looked back over his shoulder and recalled, "Come to think of it, there was one sorta confusin' spot. The trail fades out in some scree on a ridge a coupla miles back. I studied on it for quite some time without being sure where the trail was supposed to go. Still, no problem. I finally jus' pulled out my handheld GPS an' pinpointed exactly where we were."

◢

In the days after we arrived home from Kate's cancer-rediscovering surgery, we spent a great deal of time just sitting on the couch reading the paper, friends' notes, fun books, and cancer articles. I made it through a day or two without crying, but emotionally I could not, would not, accept that this disease could be happening to us. I kept hoping the whole ugly dream would end so we could get back to our lives and back to work. Everything seemed so open-ended. We felt adrift without a float, exposed with no place to hide.

For a time I saw death at every turn: a woman describing how her child would dress as "death" for Halloween; Oregon Measure 16, a proposal to make doctor-assisted suicide legal; at church the discussion of a Christian *singles'* club. At night I lay awake, unable to stop my mind from buzzing through a thousand possibilities. Every time I woke up, I listened for Kate crying because that's what caused me the greatest agony just then, the thought of Kate being frightened of death in the dark. Again I put a night-light in the bedroom to keep the room from being pitch-black. The night-light threw a pinpoint glow like a beam from far down a dark tunnel. Looking up from the bed, I wondered if death looked like this, and I felt my stomach gnawed raw.

Kate told me of her own ongoing vision of death. "I feel like a wave is pulling me away and I look on shore and see you so helpless and crying and I feel so guilty that I've ruined your life." She cried as she told me this, but then she strengthened, saying, "If it is my time, then we'll have to say we did everything we could and now it's my time and it's okay. Since there's no other choice, it has to be okay, right? We've done so much, we have to say we're happy that we've pursued our dreams, and lived the lives we wanted."

As we moved deeper into our first week home, Kate's resolve to live began to express itself. During that same period we both begrudgingly began to accept the cancer as a part of us. Given the death predictions, we couldn't deny the cancer for long if we hoped to take action against it. Accepting the cancer gave us license to start fighting it. We first visited Kate's local OB-GYN practitioner, the man who had done her cone biopsy and provided her local care. We asked what he knew about future treatment options and possible cancer cures.

The doctor looked at us with cheerless eyes and said, "Well, in your case, I don't think anyone is talking about a cure."

We left the clinic with his words and our Portland oncologist's earlier words ringing in our ears: "You could just do nothing . . . 12 to 23 months to live . . . no one is talking about a cure. . . ."

In the car, Kate looked at me solidly. Then, with stern purposefulness she said, "We clearly have the wrong doctors."

◪

With the sun starting to dip slightly, Kate and I made our way down the north side of Green Mountain toward Lewis and Clark Pass. A worn trail showed clearly at the pass, a reminder of Nez Percé travois crossings a century earlier. Curiously, Clark never made it to the pass that bears his name. Instead, it was Lewis with half of the Corps of Discovery who crossed here on their return from the Pacific. Lewis's group plied the north country in search of the northernmost tributary of the Missouri and, by extension, the young country's northernmost border from the Louisiana Purchase. Clark's group, meanwhile, explored farther south, across present-day Bozeman Pass and then down the Yellowstone River. With some seasoned skill and a healthy dollop of luck, the fragmented team somehow met near the confluence of the Missouri and the Yellowstone Rivers. The parties had traveled two unblazed paths across 500 miles of unknown land, yet arrived barely a week apart six weeks after separating.

Kate and I chose to drop off the west side of Lewis and Clark Pass down into the Alice Creek drainage to find water and a pleasant camp. Nick Williams, the CDT hiker we had met with Gordon and Sue, arrived shortly, bear bells jingling on his walking stick, massive pack on his back, and two small totes over his shoulder. Nick accepted our invitation to camp with us. He set up his tent, then joined us for a cup of tea.

We soon learned that unlike most long-distance hikers, Nick prided himself on carrying *lots* of gear. His two small totes included heaps of camera equipment, including a large telephoto lens. He had a full-size tripod lashed to his pack. He also carried a couple dozen rolls of film, explaining, "I can keep it cooler in my pack than in Gordon and Sue's van."

The camera equipment clearly brought Nick much joy. His expertise and delight in photography were equally apparent. Yet even those would be sacrificed, if necessary, to complete the CDT. "This is my year," Nick told us. "I did the AT in my 20s, the PCT in my 30s, and now the CDT in my 40s. If it gets to be too much, I'd hate it, but I'd leave the camera gear behind to finish Colorado." Handsome, mustached, and exceedingly fit, only a lack of hair hinted of Nick's ascension to middle age.

Nick also carried an ice axe, useless at this late date. "I want to hang this axe over my fireplace and say it did the entire Divide with me," he answered to our questioning looks. He carried a radio and an expensive set of solid binoculars as well. Yet with all this he also carried a titanium spoon to help minimize his pack's weight. I resisted the urge to ask if he drilled holes in his toothbrush.

"I consider myself packing psychologically light," Nick said in explanation of all the gear. "If I'm comfortable, I'm happy. If I'm happy, I hike easier. Of course," Nick deadpanned, "I used to be seven feet tall, then I took up long-distance hiking." Indeed, Nick's legs bowed out a bit.

Later that evening, we doused the fire and retired to our respective tents. A few minutes later, through the dark silence of the forest, we heard Nick's voice coming from his tent. "What is he doing?" Kate whispered to me, thinking for a moment that Nick might be a little demented. In the morning we learned that Nick wasn't talking to himself—he was listening. You see, Nick *also* carried a handheld recorder. The recorder helped him capture his thoughts throughout each day so he could better remember and record them in his journal at night.

Nick was up and mostly packed by the time Kate and I climbed out of the tent in the morning. He put in roughly 17 miles a day, so we counted ourselves lucky to have had a chance to camp with him on his shorter "townie" day. He soon hefted his pack and camera bags and bid us good hiking.

Shortly thereafter a carload of Helena folks bound for a short hike to Lewis and Clark Pass pulled up to the road's end. The previous evening Nick had predicted that everyone we would see from this point to Glacier Park would be carrying a gun. One of the men stepped out of the car and strapped on an intimidating, NYPD-worthy sidearm. "Grizzlies crawlin' all over this country," the gun toter noted a bit sheepishly after seeing our glances. "One's been botherin' the rancher a couple miles down Alice

Creek from here. I used to horse-pack folks in to this area years ago. Heard of the grizzly researchers, the Craigheads?"

An affirmative nod kept him rolling. "I packed 'em into Caribou Peak, right where you two are headin'. They used to do their studies on the griz there, griz were so plentiful."

"Thanks for the warning," we said as we shouldered our packs. Yeah, really. And thanks for ending any pretense that a few more grizzly-free nights remained. That thought was, of course, a fairy tale. A brief glance at a Montana map shows that north of where we stood, a grizzly bear—or hiker—could walk roughly 270 miles to the Canadian border and cross only two roads.

Intent on regaining the Divide, Kate and I started up the rough road along Alice Creek. We inadvertently drove 50 cattle a half mile up the drainage before they scattered into a meadow. Happily, we soon pulled away from the mindless moos and mushy cow pies. The road began to climb steadily then, crossing openings hot with morning sun. Atop the Divide, we saw a lone hiker a mile down the trail, heading south toward Lewis and Clark Pass. We felt unfortunate to have just missed an opportunity to meet another CDT hiker.

After a water and energy bar break we trudged on, now walking the knife-edge of the Divide proper. To the west and south, tree-covered mountains and barren hillsides fell away toward Lincoln. To the west and north, the majestic crown of Scapegoat Mountain showed intermittently. Closer off to the northwest, Caribou Peak, home of the Craigheads' grizzlies, commanded the view. Deep valleys, many scarred by the massive 1988 Canyon Creek fire, cut the landscape into puzzle pieces. Blue sky with wisps of high-elevation cirrus clouds arched from horizon to horizon.

Even with all the westerly beauty, it was the views north and east that held our attention. For here stretched Montana's heralded Rocky Mountain Front, an area of picket fence ridge tops and vast rock upthrusts, densely treed valleys and silent emptiness. This is the area so eloquently fictionalized by Ivan Doig. In his book *Dancing at the Rascal Fair*, Doig captures the majestic scene unfolding as one approaches the Rocky Mountain Front from the east:

Ahead was where the planet greatened.

To the west now, the entire horizon was a sky-marching procession of mountains, suddenly much nearer and clearer than they were before we entered our morning's maze of tilted hills. Peaks, cliffs, canyons, cite anything high or mighty and there it was up on that rough west brink of the world. Mountains with snow summits, mountains with jagged blue-gray faces. Mountains that were freestanding and separate as blades from the hundred crags around them; mountains that went among other mountains as flat palisades of stone miles long, like guardian reefs amid wild waves. The Rocky Mountains, simply and rightly named. Their double magnitude here startled and stunned a person, at least this one—how deep into the sky their motionless tumult reached, how far these Rockies columned across the earth.

The hem to the mountains was timbered foothills, dark bands of pine forest. And down from the foothills began prairie broader than any we had met yet, vast flat plateaus of tan grassland north and east as far as we could see. Benchland and tableland countless times larger than the jumbled ridges behind us, elbow room for the spirit. . . .

Kate and I walked on for another hour, feeling and literally being atop the world. Ahead stretched the Scapegoat and Bob Marshall Wilderness areas, places we had so often pointed to on the Montana map, places of which we had dreamed. Moving from dream to reality has always been one of Kate's strengths. To develop a singleness of purpose, to proceed despite the obstacles, to simply start, to do—these are the first steps in success. As Johann Wolfgang von Goethe once wrote,

> *Whatever you can do, or dream you can, begin it.*
> *Boldness has genius, power and magic in it.*

I have a friend who often shares a corollary to Goethe's statement: "If you don't try, you can't succeed." If Kate and I never tried to walk across Montana, even with the mental and physical challenges cancer brought to her, we would never find out if we could. If we failed, we failed. To my way of thinking, the genius and magic would still exist.

We stopped for lunch directly in front of Caribou Peak, on an alpine plateau of the Divide. A cool updraft from the valley countered the hot sun. Shortly, bear bells sounded behind us. Moments later Nick joined us for lunch, somewhat chagrined at having made a wrong turn atop Alice Creek. We thought that southbound hiker had looked familiar!

Following lunch, Nick decided to walk along with us for a while. Dropping over the next rise to a burned area on a shallow saddle, Kate suddenly halted, pointing. Ahead stood 30 elk, grazing busily on lush grasses growing under ghostly tree skeletons. Scenting us, several of the elk snorted, heads high. The band quickly bolted off the saddle, down into a grove of unburned timber.

Nick proved to be as fine a hiking partner as he was a camping mate. For miles we tackled the complexities of boots and packs, stoves and walking sticks. To Kate's and my surprise, we found that we walked at roughly the same pace as Nick. Nick, of course, carried substantially more weight, but unlike us, *he* was a bona fide long-distance hiker! True, our paltry ten miles a day paled in comparison to Nick's 17. Still, we drew strength from learning that Nick's greater distances came not so much from faster speed, but simply from putting in three or four more hours a day on the trail—day after day after day after day. . . .

◤

From Kate's journal:

> *October 12, 1994. We slept for twelve hours last night with no interruptions. The sheets felt so nice and our bed was so soft compared to those air mattress things they have at the hospital. . . . I checked the garden for strawberries. Scott got tomatoes. We picked a bunch of apples and decided to make applesauce.*
>
> *We met Scott's parents at New Morning Bakery in the afternoon. . . . I was achy sitting there and my head was getting dizzy spells. We walked around the block and then went home. I felt like my senses were being overwhelmed. I guess that's the effect of codeine.*
>
> *Scott went to talk to his dad about what he should think. He said*

his dad is the most levelheaded person he knows so he hopes to get some ideas of how to think about me having cancer and not knowing when he will lose me.

There are a million things I could do for house chores but I don't know where to start. Priorities are in a blur. Why are we making applesauce? Maybe it's therapeutic.

Talking to Terri last night was great! She is so strong and cheerful. Calling my brother was really hard. I didn't know what to say. I don't want to hurt him with talking about grim stuff.

October 13, 1994. We saw Anne and Frank driving out and Anne said she left me a card. Last night we watched a movie. . . . It was an escape to watch a movie but too scary to come back to reality. . . .

. . . I called our Corvallis doctor to ask him to take care of the HMO approvals for moving our treatment to Seattle. He said something that upset me and I got a headache and a sick stomach for an hour. "We really didn't want this to happen to you." I was silent after that. What am I supposed to say back? The statement seemed condescending toward me, as if I drew a bad card in the game I was playing and it was serious for me, but not for him.

On the cheerful side we got the kitty a Hot Catnip toy—really strong stuff—and she loved it. Also gave her a bath to get rid of that extra fur.

October 14, 1994. Scott took off early to the OHSU medical library to search for papers about studies. Terri called and asked me to walk with her and Paige on the sheep barn road. They brought me biscotti, dried fruit, and a musical instrument. Terri was good to talk to. My folks arrived shortly after that. We went on a walk in the late afternoon around the Royal Oaks route. It was the first day to really rain and it smelled good and the air was chilly. We had garden squash, and turkey, and cranberries. It hit the spot.

Scott found a bunch of abstracts of studies that used Taxol with success. He said he is encouraged by all of the things he read.

October 15/16, 1994. I felt restless so I kept busy. . . . Linda and Jeff came to visit and they were cheerful. Scott and I went for a walk in Mac Forest. Scott ran and I walked. . . . We're heading to Seattle this week to interview doctors and maybe we'll stay with Rick and Emily. . . . We'll write down our questions ahead of time to get as much information as possible. . . .

. . . I watch my dad turn to prayer for help, my mom to the experts, Scott to knowledge, others to alternative medicine, someone else to a healer, another to sound wave therapy. According to my reading, visualization is the answer. Which is the right way? I guess I'll learn about all of them to see what they can do.

Nice day today!

Less than a week after Kate left the Portland hospital, we sat in the car traveling to Seattle. We had appointments with two doctors there, Michael Smith at the Swedish Medical Center and Joanna Cain at the University of Washington Medical Center (UWMC). Dr. Smith had been our friend Pat's physician as she struggled with cervical cancer. Kate's mom had suggested Dr. Cain after seeking recommendations on OB-GYN oncologists around the western U.S. Prior to Kate's radical hysterectomy and the recent surgery, we had sought second opinions from both Dr. Smith and Dr. Cain.

Kate and I were fully committed to finding a ray of hope—not false hope, but at least a path where healing remained a possibility. Kate's current doctors seemed not to believe in the likely efficacy of the treatment options they could present us from that point forward. To live without hope for the future is no life. Yet daily Kate's will to live grew. We planned to search and learn, to try and pry open the door to hope.

We had already interviewed two oncologists in Corvallis but heard no great revelations. We'd also stopped in to visit with our friends Dick and Heidi Pattee. Years earlier they had faced death in the guise of Dick's heart valve replacement. Now they climbed mountains. Dick told us he wanted to be the three-sigma data point, the one way off the end of the survival curve that someone might mistake for an errant smudge on the plot. If nothing else, our literature searches convinced us that likewise in cancer, some people somehow survive even when cold science predicts their doom. The literature told us that medical science is in its infancy at treating and understanding cancer. We chose to see that infancy as hope.

Dr. Smith welcomed us back to his office, though he was clearly not happy at the turn of events since the last time we'd been to his office, for the radical hysterectomy interview. He suggested a combined treatment of chemotherapy and radiation, similar to treatments he had used in past cervical adenocarcinoma cases. He spoke of being aggressive, of working with experienced people, and of starting the chemo course as soon as possible. Still, Dr. Smith cautioned us, there could be no guarantee that the treatments would work.

Although we had visited Dr. Smith in person before, we had only spoken to Dr. Cain by phone. Our interview at UWMC took place in an examination room. Dr. Cain started calmly, asking me to not take notes on the computer so that we could just talk for a bit. Kate told Dr. Cain about her history: about the original mass, the cone biopsy, the radical hysterectomy, the lymphocyst, and the recent cancer-rediscovering surgery. We asked about treatments. Dr. Cain suggested a multiple-step approach, starting with a search for metastasis. If a physical exam found cancer in the lungs or lymph nodes of the clavicle, the treatment indication would change. Surgical removal of the remaining tumor would then likely be an unwarranted stress on the body, since the cancer had already metastasized. Instead, we would then pursue chemotherapy, which attacks cancer cells throughout the body. If the cancer remained in the pelvic area, Dr. Cain suggested a combination of extended field radiation and chemotherapy, followed weeks later by surgical removal of any remaining tumor and then intraoperative radiation. Unlike most of the other oncologists, Dr. Cain recommended against using Taxol since, unlike cisplatin (another chemotherapy agent), Taxol did not have a proven track record with cervical adenocarcinoma. Instead, she suggested holding Taxol as a backup treatment. She said we would monitor the response to the treatment at periodic intervals with CAT scans.

We appreciated Dr. Cain's logic process, her step-by-step approach to Kate's treatment, and her description of milestones and contingency plans. Those things alone might have led us to move our treatment north to Seattle. But it was something Dr. Cain said later—something for which

I will always give her thanks—that cemented our decision to pursue treatment with her. As with every doctor we interviewed, we asked Dr. Cain what the odds were for Kate's survival. Joanna's answer was simple and different from every other doctor with whom we spoke.

"I won't give you a prediction," she replied. Then Joanna looked directly into Kate's eyes and said, "You are a person, you are not a statistic. You are an individual, a unique person with a unique problem. We will do everything we can to get you well. We'll let the statistics worry about themselves."

Dr. Cain sent us to see Dr. Wui-jin Koh, her radiation oncology partner. Dr. Koh immediately made us feel comfortable as well. He impressed us with his ability to recall cases and distant papers from disparate topics that we had researched just that week. Dr. Koh did offer us a prediction: With Kate's health and vitality he thought she had a one in three chance of surviving. That sounded like a giant step forward to us, given that we arrived at UWMC with a one in ten expectation. Odd how little more than searching out new opinions had "improved" Kate's chance of staying alive. We grabbed hold and hung on.

◤

Nick, Kate, and I dropped into the Valley of the Moon at the base of Caribou Peak, where Kate and I decided to set up camp next to a small, unnamed lake. After reading about an eight-mile cutoff just ahead, and counting in the extra miles he had walked in the wrong direction earlier that morning, Nick decided he'd had enough for the day and would join us for another night. Later, after the dinner dishes were put away, Nick pulled out his harmonica and began to play with gusto. Suddenly three hikers marched into camp, walking sticks flashing. The men, who introduced themselves as David Patterson, Andrew Hellisell, and C.W. Banfield, asked if they could join us, and we happily agreed.

Kate and I soon discovered that David and Andrew were the two CDT walkers we had heard stories about via the hikers' grapevine in Glacier National Park. They had been snowed out on Stoney Indian Pass the day Kate and I almost started our hike. Like Nick, David and Andrew were partway through an attempt at the entire 3,100 miles of the CDT. C.W.,

who had joined the other two after Glacier, planned to hike a large section of Montana and Wyoming.

David was exceedingly thin. With a beard that hung to his chest, his
appearance was decidedly hermitlike. David started cooking and eating
and cooking and eating and then, almost crazed, began looking into his
food bag for more. "Man, that trail kicked my ass today," he said to no
one in particular. Then, looking up at the colors of the reflected sunset,
he added, "Look at that mountain. Isn't that *awe*some?"

When David learned who Nick was, he yelled out, "Nick Williams, let
me shake your hand. By God, I'm damn glad to meet you! I followed you
all the way through New Mexico! I read your trail notes all along the
way."

That started several hours of hearty trail talk. Kate and I soon learned
that long-distance hikers have a couple of umbrella organizations, the
Appalachian Long Distance Hiking Association (ALDHA) and the
American Long Distance Hiking Association–West (ALDHA–West). The
groups sponsor yearly meetings—"gatherings" in hikers' lingo—where
members join together to swap stories and gear tips. Web sites have been
established and newsletters are regularly sent out. We also learned that
the long-distance hiking community is small and well connected. David,
for example, had hiked with Walkin' Jim on the Pacific Crest Trail a year
earlier. Nick and David bantered about folks they knew in common, most
often using their trail names:

> "Have you seen Hungry Hiker?"
> "Ran into him at South Pass. . . ."
> "I heard Pieps is off, he didn't want to deal with Colorado so he
> headed for Alaska. . . ."
> "Is Lobo still on? I heard he was getting dogged. . . ."
> "Have any idea where Fiddlehead is?"
> "Last I heard, he. . . ."

Kate, David, and I did yoga on our sleeping pads, then everyone piled
into bed early. Food is the *only* thing long-distance hikers value more
than sleep. From inside their respective tents, Nick and David continued
to banter about trails, experiences, and common acquaintances. As dark

came on, Nick asked, "So David, are you planning on doing any hiking *next* summer?"

"Naw man. Nothin' big," came the muffled reply. "Nothin' over a thousand, anyway."

◢

At home in Corvallis between doctors' appointments, I sprayed the base of our peach tree with an organic treatment for leaf fungus. Looking at the tree through foggy goggles, I imagined how the chemical would be taken up by the roots and then spread quickly, systemically throughout the tree. In theory the chemical would kill the nemesis attacking our tree, but somehow allow the tree to live on and continue to bear fruit.

I shuddered as I walked into the house, thinking of the obvious parallel between the tree treatment and chemotherapy. "Chemotherapy." Talk about packaging fear into a single utterance. So much of life and death tied up in 12 simple letters. And yet that is where we had somehow arrived.

We did not willingly slide deeper into mainstream cancer treatment. Instead, during the two weeks that Kate and I interviewed new doctors, we again searched for alternatives. We spent time looking into anything and everything outside mainstream medicine that anyone suggested— prayer, nutrition, cryosurgery, vitamin therapy, the power of the mind, the healing power of electrical fields, and more.

As part of our search for alternatives, we started juicing carrots and other vegetables, with guidance from our friends Ron and Trisha. We hoped that the antioxidants available from the nutritious juices might help fight off Kate's cancer, or at least ward off other health problems to allow her immune system to concentrate all its efforts on the cancer. An hour after drinking the first glass of carrot juice, Kate ended up rolling on the bathroom floor, screaming from horrible abdominal pain. She soon withdrew into a fetal position, still quietly sobbing. "Why is the juice eating up my insides?" she moaned. "I wish it would stop!" I cried with her, leaning against the toilet as I held her. We made such a pitiful scene. Was this what dying would be like?

We had been given numerous copies of Bernie Siegel's book *Love, Medicine and Miracles,* and Kate soon started visualization techniques aimed at strengthening her immune system. Kate's journal includes drawings of good cells eating cancer cells and of the radiotherapy zapping cancer cells dead. Elsewhere, Kate drew a plethora of pink, healthy, smiling helper T-cells, all ready and eager to do battle against the unwanted cancer cells. Siegel suggested envisioning the immune system cells as something strong, white, and smart, while picturing the cancer cells as weak, ugly, and dim. Kate drew pictures in her journal of powerful white seagulls guarding a shoreline from sickly cancer cells washing up on the beach. A golden sun shines down while a thousand more seagulls fly overhead in watchful reserve.

A coworker suggested we visit a local healer in our hometown of Corvallis, a woman who had helped our coworker's son, and so we did. The healer's office was in a small, dark, nondescript building. No other patients waited in the office; the only person visible was a secretary playing solitaire on her computer. The healer introduced herself and we talked in the entranceway. She told us that she'd known of her special powers since age four, that she had once saved a drowning baby, and that she had at times been labeled a witch. She told us that when she looked at other people she saw not only their bodies but also light emitting from their chakras, the body's seven centers of spiritual energy described by the ancient religions of India.

The healer took Kate into the examination room. A massage table sat in the middle of the room. The only light came from an orange candle. "Orange is the color for the pelvic chakra," she told Kate. "I picked the candle color before you came. Though you didn't tell me what we'd be talking about, I always know the problem in advance."

The healer closed the door. Quiet, gentle sitar music started. The healer passed her hands over Kate's body, focusing on the seven chakras, hovering just above the body but not touching. She moved around the table slowly, yet purposefully. Sometimes she talked or questioned. When she finished her exam, she spoke with Kate alone.

"You are afraid of the future," the healer said to Kate. "You are treating your cancer too intellectually; you are not addressing the cancer from your heart, from your emotional chakra. You need to vent your anger.

You are panicked; your pelvic chakra is almost invisible. You feel guilty for dragging Scott into this. You two are soul mates. You are getting energy from him. But Scott must be willing to let you go or you will never be at peace. If it is truly your time—if there is nothing that can cure you—it will be okay. You will be okay and Scott will be okay. Remember, we are not given more than we can handle."

When the two of them came out to talk with me, tears began to roll down the healer's cheeks. Kate felt panicked and thought, "Why is she crying? Does she know what is going to happen to me? Can she see my death?"

"It will be difficult, painful," the healer said through watery eyes. "But I did not see death, and I am pretty good at seeing ahead. Still, what I see or don't see is not important, it is what Katie wants that is important. If she decides it is her time then my vision would change, but I don't see death now. I think Katie may have wanted me to heal her so she wouldn't have to go through with all this, but I can't do that. She has made her decision about her treatment and I would be wrong to try and change her mind."

Kate and I accepted the healer's words and tears as real and important. The words strengthened our belief that hope still existed. But we never returned to visit the healer. The whole thing seemed a little too hocus-pocus for our scientific minds. Also, I felt uncomfortable about a demonic poster hanging in the examination room and Kate was disgusted when the healer stepped outside for a cigarette in the midst of all the talk of cancer. Regardless, the healer was right about Kate having made her choice: alternatives aside, we had already decided to travel to Seattle, hoping, believing that treatment with Dr. Cain and Dr. Koh provided Kate's best shot at survival.

Our change-of-venue decision was pushed along inadvertently by our Portland oncologist himself. At the last appointment we had with him, we described what we had learned from the other oncologists we'd visited and how most of them had suggested a combined treatment of chemotherapy and radiation. The combined treatment is relatively new, we told him, and is thought to provide a synergistic benefit in fighting cervical cancer. "Yes, I know that," he replied dryly. "We all read the same journals." I'll never know if the man intended his remark to be glib. I only know that I took it that way. This isn't about your competence or ego, I wanted to scream, *this is about getting Kate well*. Kate's reaction was identical to mine. Thus though this man was an excellent oncologist, we walked out at the end of the appointment knowing we would never return.

By then we both had been given leaves of absence from our jobs with Hewlett-Packard. Thankfully, Kate was being paid via HP's long-term disability program. Our bosses and coworkers provided us with nothing but good wishes and prayers. In this instance the power of the corporation shown brightly. We will always be indebted to the people and process at HP for allowing us to quickly make the transition to focusing on Kate's health.

The insurance change of venue from Portland to Seattle did not flow so smoothly. Our HMO required us to submit a written description of why we wanted to change the location of Kate's care and why the newly proposed treatment plan was unique. Our submissions were then to be reviewed by an unknown, unseen board that we were not allowed to address.

Kate remembers, "We 'strategized' by figuring out who sat on the approval committee for the HMO. We met with each of them personally about my case, not indicating that we knew they were on the committee. We accompanied each visit with a letter spelling out the details of why the University of Washington Medical Center provided the best path for cure. We counted on the human factor and when the committee voted, I got the referral approved. It felt like a good way to start into a bigger battle."

Unstated by Kate was our commitment to travel to Seattle for treatments, regardless of the board's decision. We were fully prepared to spend all of our savings and to take out whatever loans we needed to move Kate's care north. Thankfully, the board found in our favor and granted us leave to be treated at UWMC.*

Financial and work situations thus determined, we felt blessed to have nothing left to do but spend our full energies getting Kate well.

---

* At the turn of the New Year, Kate and I changed our insurance coverage out of the HMO. Never again will we allow ourselves to be controlled by policies that don't allow patients to select their own caregivers.

◢

Our times with Dan and Sara, Gordon and Sue, Nick, David, Andrew, and C.W. provided Kate and me with a window into the long-distance hiking subculture. We had no idea so many people pursued extended backpacking trips. Gordon speculated that every year 1,500 people attempt to walk the entire AT, 500 the PCT, and 50 the CDT. On each of the trails, Gordon had guessed that roughly a tenth of those people who start succeed, with the success rate lowest on the CDT.

It's interesting to consider the motivations driving the long-distance hiker, and here let's focus just on the CDT. Goal one for most of the brethren seems to be to complete the walk in a single hiking season, come hell, high water, or deep snow. Of those who finish the CDT in a single year, hikers walking a point-to-point path from Canada to Mexico (or vice versa) claim the highest purity of execution. Jumping around with the season—assuming *every step* is walked—is still considered a continuous hike of only slightly less virtue. Hikers who "flip-flop" argue that the added purity claimed by the one-way hikers is somewhat hollow. Point-to-pointers, they note, are more likely to require road-walking stints away from the Divide to avoid surly weather.

Consider the monstrous physical and logistical demands of a journey like Dan and Sara's, the folks we met who were hiking a continuous route from north to south between the Canadian and Mexican borders. Depending on the exact route walked, the CDT runs roughly 3,100 miles. If a hiker knocks down a high average, say 20 miles a day, that's 155 days of hiking. Add a rest day every tenth day and maybe a couple of longer breaks, and the hike scratches the underbelly of six months in length. To find any kind of reasonable weather in Glacier Park means not starting the hike until June. That means walking straight through the cold fall winds and on until Thanksgiving.

Walk 20 miles, repeat eight days in a row, rest a day. Good, now repeat that process 17 more times. Freeze, roast, ache, blister, hunger. Good, now repeat for six continuous months.

Perhaps because of the demanding physical regimen, most long-distance hikers view strict adherence to the "official" CDT, the one defined in the Congressional Record, as noncompelling. Most hikers instead follow Jim Wolf's CDT guidebook, which at times deviates from the official trail but also describes routes on the approximately 30 percent of the CDT that does not yet exist on the ground. Road walking, if necessitated by bad weather, is tolerated. Wolf also describes numerous "cutoffs" that are regularly used by CDT hikers. Nowhere have I seen or heard the word "shortcut" used in connection with walking the CDT.

Like young siblings with potential, walkers like Kate and me are welcomed into the long-distance hiking crowd. They even give us a name: "big section hikers." While we big section hikers are surely part of the team, everyone understands we're still practicing on the court next door.

◪

A letter from Kate to friends and family:

November 4, 1994

Howdy,

Scott and I want to let you know what our schedule is for the next few months and where we'll be and how you can reach us and what we're doing and all that stuff.

We are going to the University of Washington Medical Center in Seattle for six weeks of treatment starting November 7th. We are renting a two-bedroom apartment on the bottom floor of a house from a woman who has set up this apartment perfectly for patients in the hospital. It has everything we need in it, so it is real easy for us to move in.

I am getting six weeks of radiation therapy (a once per day zap). During the first and fifth weeks they will administer chemotherapy (5-FU and cisplatin). I will be in the hospital Monday through Friday during those weeks. The doctors think that likely side effects will be definite tiredness, some nausea, some diarrhea, and some hair thinning. My doctors have written a paper on caffeine consumption reducing the long-term side effects from pelvic radiation. So I'm under doctor's orders to drink two Starbucks per day. Only in Seattle!

After that the default plan is to do intraoperative radiation in February, which means abdominal surgery with a douse of radiation during surgery. Hopefully all of the treatment will be done by the middle of February.

Our addresses and e-mails and phone numbers are listed below. Thanks for thinking about us. Don't be afraid to communicate. We'll let you know how things are going.

Katie and Scott

With neither of us working, Kate declared, "Let's just think of this as a fun vacation." In her journal, she made a list of 22 fun things we could do in and around Seattle. But the day we unpacked into our small apartment there, Kate quickly grew incredulous at my priorities. I filled a closet with five fly rods, waders, a vest, fly-tying gear, and a rod-wrapping jig. When she asked what I thought I was doing with all that stuff, I could only reply, "I always bring my fly-fishing gear on vacation."

"Whatever makes you feel better," Kate returned with a disbelieving shake of the head. "I suppose some people take their teddy bear wherever they go."

◪

The group rose and started folding away tents by 6:15, earlier than Kate and I generally rose, but we wanted to hike with Nick for three-quarters of a day before he bid us farewell. David, Andrew, and C.W. would be in Lincoln by nightfall. It had taken Kate and me two days to walk the same distance. By traveling farther—the three were pushing 20 miles a day—they could carry less food weight, thereby enabling and necessitating greater daily distances. Weight carried . . . daily walking distance . . . weight . . . distance—it's a balancing game all long-distance hikers play.

We marched with Nick out of the Valley of the Moon back up to the Divide, high above Bighorn Lake. Nick clicked off the names of an unending diversity of wildflowers—lupine, larkspur, buttercup, liverwort, wild rose, *Phacelia*, sticky geranium, penstemon, heather, Oregon grape, morning glory, shooting star, gentian. Full of wry, quirky wit, Nick needed no coaxing to talk and often rattled on to himself. In a quiet moment, bear bells jingling, Nick spouted, "I've got a bad case of the tinkle-itis!" In his more serious moments, Nick expressed concern that few long-distance hikers include stewardship of the trail as part of their responsibility. Nick had volunteered to maintain a section of the Appalachian Trail in his home state of Virginia and had done hundreds of hours of trail work. He guessed that the CDT might be in long-term trouble simply because few people live close enough to adequately maintain the trail.

The three of us slid down the spine of the Divide and soon dropped into land extensively burned by the Canyon Creek fire. The fire scorched a quarter of a million acres in the infamous fire summer of 1988, the year that 1.6 million acres burned in the Yellowstone ecosystem. As fires raged across the Northern Rockies, cries rang out that the land was being destroyed forever. Human beings inherently view the world through myopic, short-term spectacles. In places below us, exposed mineral soils indeed showed that much of this area had burned intensely. However, a mere ten years after the fires, lush, green grass blanketed most of the valley.

Just beyond a low saddle in the Divide, we picked up Wolf's alternate route to Blacktail Pass. Compared to the official trail, the route saved us eight miles and followed the crest of the Divide more closely. From one high vantage point, we reveled in the extended views up and down the Dearborn River valley. To the north and west a massive cliff band jutted out of the landscape like a giant picket fence, signifying our arrival in Bob Marshall country.

We parted ways with Nick at the Dearborn River, as he wanted to put in another three or four hours before nightfall. Kate and I set up camp, and activity soon surrounded us. A large guided group of horse packers erected tepees just upstream. Another horse packer, leading four gear-laden mules, rode past on the hillside above us. At the river, a mink, at first looking like a stick floating downstream, bounded out of the water ten feet from me. Fifty yards farther along a beaver tried to slap its tail at my approach, but failed because it stood on a cobbled shore.

Kate and I spent the next couple of nights camped not far upstream along the Dearborn, opting for a day and a half of rest and some time fishing. The fish proved enthusiastic. They came to the fly endless times—mostly wild cutthroats with deep yellow slashes and heavy, black spots—and all caught on highly visual, "the-bigger-the-better" type dry flies. The fish held not so much in pocket water behind large boulders but instead in deep, rocky runs. All fought with vitality. One of the bigger cuts raced down a long rapid and then under a log. It took me a full minute to revive the fish and thank it for the battle.

Our rest day camp was idyllic—near the creek, in a big grassy opening with the occasional large pine, with a campfire in the meadow and the tent in a sheltered grove. While I fished, Kate rested and read in camp with three neighborly whitetail deer. Once Kate heard a screech. Later, together, we heard the screech again. The cry pierced the air like nothing we'd ever heard. For a moment we thought of a screech owl, then a mountain lion, then perhaps one of the deer being killed. Kate thought the second screech sounded from lower, closer to the river and nearer us. What was going on? I piled rocks and a large stick by the tent, but the sound never recurred.

◰

Drip . . . drip . . . drip . . . watching the drops of chemotherapy fall from the IV bag . . . drip . . . drip . . . drip. . . . We were sitting at the crossroads of life and death, a milestone beyond which nothing would be the same; and yet there, sitting quietly in her hospital bed, sat Kate, looking exactly like her healthy self. "I looked at the bag of chemo," Kate recalls, "and tried to visualize how it would help me."

Sun streamed in the window. Drip . . . drip . . . drip. . . . For hours everything was normal—so normal, in fact, that when Ellen arrived and said, "Well this is boring, you're not even throwing up or anything," we could all smile.

By dinner, Kate was bored and wanted to walk around the hospital. "No problem," she decided. "Maybe I'm one of those people who doesn't get sick."

We ended up at the hospital cafeteria. Suddenly with no warning nausea overwhelmed her and Kate threw up. I cleaned up as best I could and we quickly started back for Kate's room, pushing the IV pole ahead.

Thus began six days of agony. Ninety-six hours of 5-FU (fluorouracil, a drug that makes radiation more effective), with an early-on two-hour infusion of cisplatin. Daily radiation. Vomiting. Blood tests. Retching. Bloating with IV fluids. Endless coughing. By the third day, Kate's 32nd birthday, she said she couldn't take it anymore. She begged me to get her out of the hospital. I could only hold her hand and look on in despair. By the fourth day, Kate was essentially unconscious when I wheeled her down for her daily radiation treatment.

"I couldn't lift my chin off my chest," Kate remembers, "and I couldn't tell the radiation technician that she was pulling the IV out of my arm when she moved my IV pole away from the field of radiation."

Vomiting . . . medication . . . nausea . . . new medication . . . vomiting . . . Idle and in agony for Kate, I charted the times between each new medication and the next vomiting episode, hoping to find some correlation that would help us pick the right anti-nausea medicine. I came up with nothing. There would be nothing but misery for Kate.

From Kate's journal:

> *November 14, 1994. I'm home from the hospital now. Today I felt good as I woke up. But when I took a shower I felt really bad. Dr. Raymond was analytical and measured blood pressure and pulse sitting and standing and the pulse raced and the BP dropped. He said I was way low on fluids. He said I should get an IV with saline. No way! They missed two times before finding a vein in the hospital and I already have enough bruises. The other option I have is to drink 3 liters of Gatorade today to rehydrate, so that's what I'm doing. I have had enough of needle torture. I can't even think about that now.*
>
> *I can't even think about going back in for more chemotherapy. It was the most hopeless feeling I ever had. It was horrible. I puked for 6 days. I couldn't eat and drink. Every time I peed Scott would have to unplug the IV pole and roll me in. Walking was so dizzying. My legs felt like sticks to balance on but with no muscles to use. The IVs had pumped 20 extra pounds into me so I felt totally bloated. My loose sweats were skintight. My face was bloated.*
>
> *I remember my parents being in the room a lot. Bill came to visit but I only remember his face as a blur. I don't even remember last Wednesday or Thursday.*

Dr. Cain said I was having a longer time than normal coming out of it. I stayed in the hospital 2 extra days. It is going to take a lot of forgetting to make myself go for another round of chemo. None of the seven anti-nausea drugs worked.

When I got home I lay on my back by the heater and moaned. My stomach and throat and mouth cramped and burned when I drank anything. My mouth had big puffs of swelled lining that stuck out. My nose started bleeding and wouldn't stop when I blew it. My eyes could not focus quickly for the whole chemo so when I walked I could only look at the ground. I couldn't flash a look at a person who came in the room to say "Hi." When I rolled over and changed my position I puked or got a wave of nausea. I tried eating some ice cream and it came up like a stick of half-melted butter. It was so gross I think it will be one of those food experiences I'll never forget. I doubt I'll eat rich ice cream again.

I talked to Pat Davidson. She had listened to her tapes from 4 years ago that she made during treatment. I thought she had the same treatment I'm having but she had more! She had 4 chemotherapies total. I don't know how she could have gone back for another one after knowing what they were like. Her experiences were very similar to mine as far as misery and anti-nausea drugs not working. It was really good to talk to her. . . .

My goal today is to get fluids in! I'll feel good tomorrow!

◪

Bouncing up the trail the morning after our rest day, we passed through a cooler burn: instead of denuded ground, dead or simply scorched trees still stood and thousands of knee-high lodgepole pines blanketed the forest floor. Showy fireweed and bear grass rose above the new pines. Life burst from the "dead" forest. Ahead, expansive views of Crown Mountain beckoned, visible because of the burn.

A horseback rider and dog waited at the trail cutoff to Straight Creek Pass. Janelle Rieger, a slim woman, wore the khaki greens of a Forest Service backcountry ranger. A long ponytail hung from under her hat. When she pulled off her sunglasses, Janelle revealed a tan and friendly face. After a brief conversation, she delayed the start of her patrol into Halfmoon Park and invited us to her cabin.

At the cabin, Janelle offered us cookies and spring water lemonade. As we greedily dug in she laughed, "You hikers always eat so much, I can't believe it." Not wanting to disappoint her, I ate a dozen Double Stuf Oreos and a half dozen substantial slabs of cheese.

The Welcome Creek cabin, vintage 1934, had a small solar panel that ran a radio ("Sure, I get Choteau and Augusta"), an outhouse, and a spring. Janelle kept the cabin clean, sparse, and pleasant. The Forest Service had saved the Welcome Creek cabin from the Canyon Creek fire by horse packing in a pump, gasoline, and an asbestos tarp, then continuously sprinkling down the roof.

"Some people want to tear these cabins down," Janelle said, turning to a topic that clearly held some emotion for her. "I think maybe they're pushing the concept of wilderness too far. These buildings are historic, built roughly a trail's day apart. People don't realize that the trail crews use them, or that someone in real trouble could break in if they had to. I get lots of people in here who can't even read a map or use a compass."

Janelle brought her own horses into the wilderness and wasn't terribly upset by the big pack trains of dudes. She had registered a previous day's group as 24 horses, 13 people. "Doesn't two horses per person seem like a lot of wear on the local ecology?" I asked.

"For some folks, that's the only way they can get in here," she replied. "And don't forget, those people go back to the city and become wilderness supporters because of what they've been able to see and experience."

For several years Janelle had been coming to Welcome Creek for June through September. The rest of the year Janelle and her husband run a ranch in Ismay, a town far off on Montana's eastern plains. "Being from Wise River," she said, sliding the cheese block a little closer my way, "where my dad was Forest Service, growing up on the Anaconda–Pintler and all, if I couldn't get my fix of mountains in once a year, I couldn't live out there on the ranch. Besides, my husband likes the money; it helps out for fixing things back home."

Janelle described how her town of Ismay once voted to call itself "Joe," after then–Kansas City quarterback Joe Montana. It seems a Kansas City disc jockey decided that Joe Montana really needed to have a town

named after him. So the disc jockey called Ismay's town clerk and suggested they make the change for the duration of the 1993 football season.
Ismay was at the time Montana's smallest incorporated town, so when
the town clerk, the two city council members, the mayor, and a handful
of locals gathered, few of the town's twenty-two residents were not in
attendance.

"Why not be called 'Joe'?" was apparently the group's consensus. In
return for the name change, the disc jockey offered to fly the town clerk,
the mayor, and the mayor's family to a Chiefs' game. Sensing he had the
media in a stranglehold, the wily town clerk held out for, and received, a
better deal—a trip to Kansas City for Ismay's entire populace!

◢

Kate's brother, Bill, flew in from Colorado to be with her during part of
the chemotherapy treatment. Living in different states, Bill and Kate had
not seen each other since we had learned of the recurrence of Kate's cancer. Now face-to-face at the hospital, they would still effectively be apart.
Even days after the chemotherapy wore off, Kate barely remembered Bill's
visit.

Many times during his several day stay, Bill stood next to Kate's bed,
looking down in disbelief at his sister's bloated, semiconscious body.
Even when he left to return home to his wife Chris and our niece Corrie,
disbelief continued to shade his face.

"Finding out about Kate's cancer made me angry at the world," Bill
has told me since. "I could not find a reason or purpose for it to have happened. To me Kate is uniquely special and precious—my little sister. She
always seemed to be doing the right things in life.

"Knowing that good people sometimes suffer is a real anomaly for
me. I was young when my mother was very ill in the hospital. I really
have no concept of how grave that situation was, only what I have been
told. Kate's illness seemed so unreal to me that I was yelling out for
Karmic justice."

Kate and Bill share a love for the outdoors, for fun, and for the eso-
teric. In 20 years, I don't think I've ever heard a cross word between
them. "When I was visiting Kate in the hospital," Bill went on to say, "I

was feeling tremendous awe and grief. I realized that her path had fogged. She was now on her own journey into something only she could understand. I was angry, but at the same time frustrated, questioning whether she had made the right choices. I mean that possibly she had given in to what the doctors had diagnosed too readily. I wanted her to make irrational choices. *Just don't believe it, use your mind to overcome the cancer, find an alternative!* At the time I was foolishly thinking that everyone involved was being seduced by fear.

"I have now come to understand how brave her decisions were along the way," Bill concluded. "I now see her in a different way. I try to know her through her experiences, as if she has been to places in her mind that I have not. Events like these make me wonder just how much control we have in our lives. Many of my illusions about my little sister and my life have changed."

◪

Kate and I left Janelle and padded up Welcome Creek to gentle Straight Creek Pass. Ahead was a long, straight valley with much unburned forest. After a night at Cigarette Creek, we walked out along Straight Creek, heading for the small dude ranch at Benchmark where Kate's parents, a resupply box, and a couple of days off awaited us. Partway down to Benchmark, a large buck mule deer, still in velvet, stood in midstream. He stepped forward boldly, caught wind of us, then turned and bounced off into the forest.

Past the deer, Kate had a bad spate with her bowels. As she hurriedly threw off her pack, she almost fell off a steep section of the trail. When we were hiking again I stupidly asked why the bowel fits had not happened during the two days we'd hiked with Nick. Kate blew up. "Do you think I'm making this up? It's so hard. You could never do what I have to do!" she yelled this in anger and in truth. Kate started to cry and, throwing my arm off, marched away.

Farther along I was able to stop her, but still she cried. "What are you thinking?" I asked.

"Nothing, I'm just feeling sorry for myself."

"You are the toughest person I have ever known," I said, choking up with the truth of my statement.

We walked out the bottom of the drainage and into the small set of tourist cabins at Benchmark. The place seemed wholly Western, wholly, happily, disorganized. The propane tank for our stove was empty, so I found tools and replaced it myself. The box springs in our room proved so flimsy that Kate and I would later have to tether ourselves to the edges of the mattress to keep from crashing together in the middle. Still, after a hot shower and the arrival of Kate's parents with a carload of food, we rested happily for two days.

Come to think of it, the springs on the bed couldn't have been too bad—we slept soundly through two nights of black bear assaults on the garbage cans outside. On the first night, our neighbors lost a whole watermelon they'd set on the front porch to cool. On the second night, we "bear-ified" our cabin complex and lost nothing. Another neighbor fared poorly, however, losing an entire case of beer from the back of his pickup. Every can had been neatly punctured by a suds-loving bruin.

◪

Kate and I had been blessed to find an apartment near the University of Washington Medical Center that two good people, Linda Hein and Glen Reese, rented out only to cancer patients. They had set up the apartment fully so that UWMC patients undergoing treatment could move in and immediately start focusing on getting well. The day we arrived in Seattle, Kate and I had attacked a walnut torte left at the apartment by our friend Emily Tidball. Now, back at the apartment after the chemotherapy, it would be days before Kate could eat more than a small baked potato.

We hunkered down in the tiny apartment and our life took on a regular pattern. Daily we went to the cancer center for Kate's radiation. Almost daily, it seemed, blood draws showed Kate's red blood cell count to be low and her immune system depressed. These deficiencies likely occurred because chemotherapy attacks the cells in the bone marrow. To combat these problems, Kate received blood transfusions and G-CSF, an expensive compound that stimulates white blood cell production. The days and the radiation treatments continued, but soon Dr. Cain postponed the second round of chemotherapy due to Kate's low white blood cell count. Still, ever and always, day after day, we came for the radiation treatments.

One night, huddled deep into the apartment, Kate and I cried together, just remembering the agony of chemotherapy. Kate talked about how tough it was for her to see little kids being treated for cancer, how they were too young to know that life holds good and happy moments, too.

From Kate's journal, during the middle of the radiation treatments:

> *December 4, 1994. We did lots of fun things during the latter part of November. I'm growing stronger after chemo and the radiation side effects are not so noticeable, except for diarrhea. My hair is thinning rapidly. . . .*
>
> *Joan and Jon and baby Katie came down from Nelson, B.C. They were fun to have around. They fixed organic meals, had great ideas, and were uplifting. We rode the ferry across Puget Sound with Rick & Em and baby Kevin and tooled around the town of Winslow. . . .*

Along with friends, a medical team coalesced around Kate during those six weeks of outpatient radiation treatment, good people who began to know Kate and care for her and truly connect with her. We talked with Dr. Cain and Dr. Koh about milestones and treatment-changing decisions. They listened when we talked about papers I'd read in the library and were not offended when we asked them to defend a choice in light of research we had turned up. They made decisions during our checkups, discussing the options, balancing the risks, in front of us, *with* us. When Drs. Cain and Koh asked if we wanted to take extra time off at Thanksgiving to be with our families, we asked Dr. Koh if the radiation treatment worked best if no breaks existed. He said he would have to check the studies, but he thought that yes, continuous treatments would be best.

That information in hand, we stated simply, "We're here to get well. We'll be back Friday, the day the Cancer Center reopens."

Kate's team grew from its center. Almost daily, we talked with Jim Raymond, Dr. Koh's chief resident. Jim was a man our age, a former engineer and a mountain climber, a man who unabashedly shared his knowledge and—as important—his friendship and good nature. Carol Mickley and Katy Jusenius, two of the lead oncology nurses, often hugged Kate when they greeted her. We'd also been blessed by connecting with Jana Ghosn, the lead floor nurse on 6NE who had looked after Kate through the chemotherapy week. And the list went on: radiation techs and receptionists and the nurses who drew Kate's blood. So many people would see Kate in the hallways, ask how things were progressing, and wish her well.

Our team had its shady elements as well. We had heard from an acquaintance that smoking pot was the only way to survive chemotherapy. Neither Kate nor I smoke pot, yet we agreed that having some on hand for the next round of chemotherapy might help, given the agony Kate experienced during the first round.

One night we received a comically cryptic phone message on the machine at our apartment: "Hi this is . . . uh . . . uh . . . well, you know who this is. Anyway, I just wanted to tell you that I left the . . . uh . . . er . . . stuff, you know, the *stuff* hidden in the plant on your front doorstep. I sure hope it helps. I can get you some more . . . er . . . stuff if you want. Just let me know, okay. See ya, I'm leaving town now."

Giff and Ellen spent most of the treatment time in Seattle with us. One night they went for dinner at a Chinese restaurant. At the end of the meal Giff broke open his fortune cookie. The slip of paper inside, which Kate later taped in her journal, read:

The Physician Heals, Nature Makes Well

SIX

◣

At Cliff's Edge

The man told us, " . . . No one will know if you live or die out there."
Those words stayed with me all day as we moved across the featureless sand hills,
following the compass. No one would know if we lived or died. No one.
There was no one here but Marinetta and me, and we hardly
counted as separate people anymore.

MICHAEL ASHER
Impossible Journey

A BOUT A MILE into the Bob Marshall Wilderness, Kate's parents turned to bid us goodbye. Unsure as ever about the wisdom of her daughter's journey, Ellen jokingly offered us a free month's lodging anywhere we wanted if we just would quit the hike. We declined, hugged them, then started off down the track as Giff and Ellen headed back to the trailhead.

The trail moved through lowland lodgepole forest and often ran as wide as a two-lane highway. Although sometimes muddy, the tread showed evidence of substantial efforts by the U.S. Forest Service and a group of professional outfitters. Then, after four or five miles, we came to what must be one of the biggest public works projects in our national wilderness system, an enormous wooden stock bridge spanning the West Fork of the Sun River. If we hadn't guessed it from the ratio of horse trailers to unattached cars back in the parking lot, the bridge confirmed that we would see far more horse packers than hikers in the days ahead.

Ellen's offer sounded pretty good a few miles past the big bridge. We paused for lunch and to let a horse train of dudes pass. Farther on, high above the river, we started around a corner toward an open glade. I stopped, still behind the last of the trees and whispered, "Bear." We peered through the branches long enough to see a blonde animal— honey blonde. We could not discern if the animal was a black bear or grizzly, but decided to be prudent and backtrack to a campsite we had seen two miles earlier. This was the bear that would later join Kate at the campfire.

I should explain about the campfires. To save weight, Kate and I had been carrying a lightweight stove that required no fuel, but rather burned pinecones, small sticks, and the like. We were finding the stove highly unlikable; too small for easy fuel feeding, it also made sooty messes of our pot and itself. Even before Lincoln, we had started cooking over an open fire because we could more easily control the temperature. At Lincoln, we bought a small baking pan to protect our pot and sent the stove home. We chose our fire locations with care and steadfastly reclaimed those that weren't built in existing fire pits.

Still, fire carries a smell, and the blonde bear that did the do-si-do with Kate appeared shortly after we started our fire that night. When the bear finally ambled off up the hill, we decided it best to vacate the area to better avoid a nighttime encounter. We doused the fire, retrieved the food, and then after hurriedly packing headed back up the trail in the opposite direction of the bear's tracks. That was at 8 P.M. Past 10, as we began to wonder about the intelligence of wandering the woods at night, we saw a fire below the trail. Four college kids from Missoula allowed us to pitch our tent with them. The kids mentioned that the backcountry ranger had stopped earlier to warn of a grizzly spotted that day on the trail.

The ranger, Macon, dropped back down from Indian Creek Guard Station early in the morning, intent on learning about bear trouble in the valley. Macon woke us in the tent and interviewed Kate as we lay in our shared sleeping bag. Macon wore a cowboy hat and as he knelt at the door of the tent I couldn't help but notice his massive calf muscles. As Kate described the encounter, Macon made notes, clucking disapprovingly upon hearing that the bear had approached the fire, had not run away, and had shown aggression by growling. Kate described the bear as a blonde black bear. Macon said that the horse outfitters just in front of us had reported seeing a young *grizzly* bear in the same meadow where we first encountered it, and that the bear had approached their group without fear. The horse packers had expressed concern about the two hikers shortly behind them—us—but had not sent anyone back as an expression of that concern.

Resting on her elbows, Kate wound down her bear story, finishing, oddly, with, "And he was so cute. I was scared but also kept thinking, 'This is the cutest bear I've ever seen.'"

After Macon had his hands around our story, he pressed Kate a second time, "So you think it might have been a blonde black bear rather than a young griz?"

"I don't *think* so, it *was* a black bear." Kate set her chin. "It stood right next to me and I got a plenty good look at it." She and I had talked about the bear's identification on our late night walk up the valley. I could remember a black bear profile on our first sighting, but when it snarled at us over its shoulder the face seemed more dished out, like a griz. And there was that honey blonde coat. Still, Kate remained strong in her conviction, so I said nothing.

Later that morning, a big group of Scouts passed as we made our way up the declining waters of the West Fork of the Sun. The Scout leader, who carried a sidearm *and* bear spray, stopped to tell us they were on a 50-miler. Horse packers had carried in the majority of the Scouts' gear and food, he said without embarrassment, including fresh halibut from Alaska. I asked if trout would have been too easy and he laughed good-naturedly. But when I told the Scout leader I reckoned we only did 33 miles on my own Scouting 50-miler, his look turned hangdog and he muttered something about needing to catch up with the boys.

Halibut! The big Scout group helped prove Macon's two principles for safe camping in bear country. First, avoid using fire pits at existing sites. Big groups often carry food backpackers would never consider. By using an existing pit we might be sending out the smell of bacon grease that someone had dumped a previous night. And with only two people instead of a group to contend with, a bear would be much less reluctant to enter our camp and investigate the smell. Principle number two: Camp off the trail. Since bears and other wildlife use the trails, camping off trail helps avoid inadvertent nighttime contact.

Kate and I hiked on and up through dense forest, then decided to cook dinner for lunch to avoid needing a fire near the camp that night. Although our packs weighed less because we'd begun cooking over fires, more and more we missed having our white gas stove. The daily convenience provided by a stove began to overshadow our initial concern about weight. Plus, as Macon had suggested (and as we now believed), to a human-habituated bear, the smell of a fire alone provides a sufficient call to dinner. We both looked forward to picking up our backpacking stove when we returned to the car at East Glacier.

◪

Kate almost panicked and jumped off the table during the last of her radiation treatments. The machine remained on for much longer that day than any day during the rest of the six weeks. Dr. Koh had narrowed the field and increased the time for the final boost.

As we departed the Cancer Center, everyone congratulated Kate on being finished with her treatments. Several people gave her big, warm hugs. So many times that week we had heard, "Boy, it seems like you've been here forever . . . what a great milestone . . . what are you going to do next?"

We appreciated these people's support and good thoughts, but they were suddenly no longer part of our reality. In truth, they had always been just momentary stepping-stones on our crossing to health. Being immersed in treatment had totally absorbed us and now, abruptly, we were done. By the time we sat alone in the car, in the quiet parking garage, Kate began to cry.

"What *do* we do next?" she said through her tears.

I held her and quietly said all that I could say. "Now we live."

◪

Late one afternoon hints of the famous Chinese Wall began to show through the trees ahead. The short glimpses of vertical limestone recalled the Rimrocks of my hometown of Billings, Montana, but at several times the magnitude. Kate and I pulled into a place to camp, secluded from all but the top of the Wall by tall pines, off the trail with no fire rings in sight, but able to hear the noise from an outfitter's camp about a quarter mile away. We ate our lunch for dinner, went for a short walk, then crawled into the tent at 7:15 to read aloud to each other. The Chinese Wall acted as a giant sunscreen; our sunset had long ago passed.

Soon a voice outside hailed us. It was Dale, the lead wrangler for the outfitted group camped nearby. Dale had his 15-year-old son in tow. We had talked to the two of them earlier in the day. Dale's pack string—an impressive set of large mules—ran clean and smooth as they passed us. Both Dale and his son wore cowboy hats just as they had when we'd seen them earlier, but Dale no longer carried his sidearm.

Dale introduced his son, saying, "This is the boy's first trip." Then, as he dropped to the ground to sit, Dale said with a smile, "By damn a year off. Walkin' the Divide—that's smart. Now that's somethin' I'd do." I climbed out of the tent to sit with the two wranglers while Kate talked from the tent's door.

Dale's mules brayed in the distance, and he motioned toward his camp, saying, "Some of these people we got with us been with some bad outfitters before. They can't believe we brush the stock, look for saddle sores, treat our animals right."

The boy watched Dale closely. When Dale spat, the boy spat.

We talked about horse packing for a while, and then I asked about llamas. Dale didn't care for llamas much. "I always send a rider in front of me to warn others on a tight trail that my train is comin'. Hell," he said acerbically, "llama packers'll never do that."

If llamas acted as the kindling, then my mention of forest fires provided the fuel for Dale to get truly worked up. "This is my country here, and I don't want it ruined. They got so damned many rules—let it burn, my ass! Hell, elk need the deep forest! And what about the jays? I say let eight or ten thousand acres burn, then put it out. Some of this country will never come back—ever!"

Dale reached down, plucked a piece of grass, and stuck it in his mouth. The boy repeated Dale's action precisely. Looking up, Dale turned to grizzlies. "You track a griz in this country in the snow and you've got yourself a heap o' trouble. He'll double back on ya or just lay up for ya. A griz jumped one of my hunters last year. Shot him with a 300 mag at 12 feet."

Dale was a fit man, no glasses, maybe 45 years old. Grizzlies, elk hunting, and the Bob all clearly impassioned him, making the muscles of his neck strain. "Things have changed since we stopped huntin' griz. Used to be you'd shoot and griz'd scatter. Now they all come a runnin' 'cause they think ya got somethin' down. I've had 'em face off with me, snortin' and twirlin' and jumpin' up and down. One time I fired my pistol into the ground in front of one *four* times! Next shot I swore I was gonna kill 'im. Had a guy with a 300 backin' me."

Dale crossed his legs. "This no huntin' business ain't no fair to people like you neither, 'cause the bears ain't scared of you like they used to be. Do you know that they kill more bears for 'administrative' purposes now than we ever took hunting them?* What harm were we doin'?"

When Dale paused, his son spoke for the first time, unwarranted

---

* Dale's concept seemed intriguing, so I checked with bear biologists Arnold Dood and Helga Pac at Montana Fish, Wildlife, and Parks. Arnold noted that such a simplistic statement would be almost impossible to conclusively prove from the data since variables such as food crop, people pressure, and habitat loss also come into play. He noted that hunters often talk incorrectly about the "negative conditioning" benefit that hunting provides. As Arnold pointed out, animals killed by hunting clearly can't pass on that "negative conditioning" to their offspring. A selective pressure, however, does exist. In other words, hunters will slowly select against animals that are not afraid of humans or that spend lots of daylight time in the open.

Helga provided me with grizzly mortality rates for the Northern Continental Divide (essentially from Missoula and State Road 200 north to the Canadian border) for dates before and after legal hunting ended in 1991. That data shows that in the eight years prior to the 1991 hunting ban, 101 grizzlies died from known and probable human causes, including 34 bears killed by hunters and 16 killed for management control. "Management control" is a wildlife professional's euphemism for killing "problem" bears, for example, those that tear up cabins or prey on livestock. In the eight years after the ban, 103 grizzlies died from known and probable human causes, including 0 by hunting and 36 killed for management control reasons. Ignoring the complexities Arnold spoke of, the data certainly seems to lean in favor of one of Dale's contentions: there's been a shift from hunting mortalities to management control mortalities.

It is not as clear whether the grizzlies have become less wary of humans since the ban on hunting. For example, self-defense-related mortalities stayed essentially the same in the eight years before and after the end of hunting (6 versus 7, respectively). Elk and deer hunters are often involved in those self-defense deaths. The best summary statement I heard for the situation came from Mark Haroldson, another grizzly researcher: "Whether you can legally hunt for griz or not, anytime men, guns, and bears come in close proximity, bears will be killed."

wisdom sounding in the boy's voice, "Too damn many bears in this country right now, I'd say."

When we told Dale about Kate's run-in with the honey blonde bear, and of her certainty that it was a black bear, Dale countered with, "Coupla yearling, very blonde grizzlies got trapped near Choteau last year. They were released on the South Fork of the Sun. Coulda been one of them. A young griz, 'specially a poor one, might not have much of a shoulder hump."

Kate's bear definitely did not look "poor," but the question continued to intrigue me: Had Kate stared down a grizzly?

Dale and his son soon departed, but Dale's stories stayed with me and did little to ease my growing sense that the Bob really was griz country. While we knew this fact, of course, the small detail about grizzlies no longer being hunted somehow had fallen through the cracks. Suddenly all those "you'll-be-lucky-to-see-a-griz-in-the-Bob" stories rang hollow.

Sleep came. Past midnight I went from dead slumber to instantly awake. My eyes opened wide. I did not move, did not even lift my head, did not even blink. Heavy breathing outside the tent. Then a snort. Then another. So close! I nudged Kate awake and whispered, "Grab your bear spray! Get the cap off!"

"What!?" and in that instant she also floated on adrenalin. We both lay on our stomachs, elbows under us, holding our bear sprays in hand and tilting our heads to the noises.

The raspy breathing continued. Now something clawed the ground . . . so incredibly close. And then the guy line on the tent snapped as the snorting beast tripped, shaking our shelter. Then a louder snarl! My heart climbed into my throat as we began to live out the worst grizzly horror, the one with a million-to-one odds—the attack in the tent!

A minute went by and still the snorts and raspy wheezes continued. Breathing became extremely difficult with my heart in my throat. Then Kate, in a whisper, said, "It might be a deer. They like salt and I peed over there."

"No listen, it's in our packs," I said, motioning with my bear spray.

"Shhh. I don't think that's the packs. Careful, just don't spray us with that thing, okay?"

In another minute, we couldn't take the snorts any longer. In a whis-

pered plan we decided to make noise together. "Okay, ready? One
. . . two . . . three . . . HEY, HEY, HEY, HEY! GET OUT OF HERE!!"

We listened, straining, to learn if we'd saved ourselves or clanged the
dinner bell. The noises stopped . . . silence . . . then a footfall . . . then
another. Farther away? Yes, but only a step or two. A pause . . . then rasp-
ing, hot, wet breath again. Then for the first time an odd clacking noise—
a grizzly popping its jaws in anger?

Suddenly everything went silent. Then a loud, fast, repetitive thud.
"What's that?" Kate whispered urgently. "What *is* that?" Terror sounded
in her voice for the first time.

I looked at her through the darkness, barely able to breathe.
"Ah . . . it's my . . . ah . . . my heart beating." Even during the most
strenuous interval training, I could have never made it beat so hard.

I felt Kate's incredulous look through the darkness. Letting out a big
breath, she whispered, "I still think it might be a deer."

More pawing and snorts then, this time definitely farther away. We
could stand it no longer, we concurred, we had to look. I'd already said
the Lord's Prayer; what else could we do? To wait still longer, after two or
three minutes of raw fear of the unknown, was unthinkable. And so bear
sprays in one hand, flashlights in the other, we knowingly broke the
code. The tent, flimsy though it be, can be the last psychological obstacle
to a bear attacking a camper in the night. By opening the door we would
create an encounter; we would eliminate that final barrier.

I unzipped the tent. On the ground two feet to the right was the
depression and loose dirt of a fresh dig mark. Ahead, at the edge of the
trees, a large . . . mule deer pogo-ed away, the thud of hooves rather than
the padding stillness of paws moving into the darkness.

It took only a shudder and one deep sigh of relief before Kate descended on me, pounding me on the back, "Your heart! Your heart, for
God's sake! That's the only time I was scared, when I heard your heart!"

I could see it all too clearly. Front page headline, *Helena Independent
Record:*

BACKPACKER DIES IN THE BOB
Heart Attack Thought to be Brought on by
Mule Deer Encounter

◪

Kate's initial radiotherapy and chemotherapy may have been complete, but her treatments were far from over. Drs. Cain and Koh, who at the time were writing a national protocol for treating recurrent cervical cancer like Kate's adenocarcinoma, believed that a radiation dose of 5,400 rads was insufficient to eradicate Kate's cancer. However, they felt confident that the cancer would be eliminated at 7,000 rads. Unfortunately, they also knew that the bowel could not absorb that much radiation without irreparable damage. Thus they had built Kate's radiation treatment plan around a 5,000- to 6,000-rad external beam exposure. During that treatment they had had Kate lie on foam blocks to wedge her bowel as much as possible out of the field of radiation. The doctors' plan then called for a six-week wait followed by surgical removal of the remaining tumor combined with internal radiation—meaning radiation given with the body cavity open. The latter process, known as intraoperative radiation treatment (IORT), would allow the tumor to be exposed to the remaining radiation dose (to make 7,000 rads total) without the risk of bowel involvement.

Two or three rounds of chemotherapy had originally been planned for the six weeks of radiation plus a potential final chemo round just prior to the IORT surgery. Kate's immune system was so overwhelmed by the first chemotherapy, however, that Drs. Cain and Koh had postponed, postponed, and finally abandoned all thoughts of even one more chemotherapy round. Kate's white blood cell count, platelet count, and hematocrit (the ratio of red blood cells to plasma, or whole blood) fell alarmingly low and did not recover following the one round of chemo she did have. During the weeks she received external beam radiation, Kate received growth-stimulating injections for her immune system, several blood transfusions, and iron supplements. I gathered strength from the thought that if her bone marrow had taken that much of a beating, the cancer must surely be suffering.

A lot of other things also suffered during those six weeks of radiation treatment. Shortly after the chemotherapy week, Kate's hair began to fall out in clumps. Initially, Kate agonized over the hair loss. Later, while at Nordstrom's and Seattle's Pike Street Market, Kate's parents and I bought her hats that she would wear for months. Perhaps because Kate's hair has always been so thick, it did not all fall out. Instead, throughout that winter she lived with wispy hair, perhaps a quarter head full.

Kate worried that I was suffering, too, and she expressed concern about the stress I had to shoulder in caring for her. All I could think of was the smallness of my trials compared to what she'd been enduring. But in truth I fared poorly those weeks. I stupidly broke a kitchen floor tile in our rented apartment, locked my keys in the car, started down the freeway the wrong way, and eventually caused an automobile accident in which no one, thankfully, was hurt.

During the six weeks of Kate's radiation, our major piece of sanity— aside from Kate's folks and a visit or two from out-of-town friends—came from regular visits, dinners, and walks with our friends Rick and Emily Tidball. We'd met Rick and Emily back in Boulder, around the same time Kate and I met at the University of Colorado. Rick, like me, was a graduate student in chemical engineering. Emily worked for IBM. We formed a happy friendship in Boulder, one that continued when they moved to California and then later to the Seattle area.

Rick and Emily shared our excitement about a midtreatment CAT scan that showed that Kate's tumor was shrinking. They listened and helped us logically talk through each possible new treatment idea. Emily, who had most recently worked in the biomedical field, provided a solid wall to bounce thoughts off. Rick brought a levelheadedness to our situation that I was absolutely incapable of achieving. Most important, much of the time the four of us didn't speak of health at all. After endless days living out our hospital identities, Rick and Emily allowed Kate and me to reclaim our own identities. We drew strength from every interaction with them.

◤

Dale had his group of dudes up, packed, saddled, and riding away by the time Kate and I climbed out of the tent in the morning. As he rode past us, Dale said the mule deer had bothered their camp in the middle of the night as well. He had swatted it on the rump with a branch.

Starting up through the trees, Kate and I soon began to see the

Chinese Wall in all its magnificence. The massive rock dominates the trail like a battleship dominates a wooden dock. This endless reef of sheer limestone is in places a thousand feet tall. We could not take in the Chinese Wall's height and width in a single glance. Rather than simply looking at the Wall, one must survey it, up and down, far and near, to the horizon line or to the half moon rising over a high point. If the Great Wall of China is a wonder of man, then the Chinese Wall of Montana is certainly a wonder of God.

Though this is reputed to be the most popular place in the Bob, after Dale's group left us at the southern end, Kate and I would walk the length of the wall, 13 miles, without seeing another soul. We walked and gawked, feeling so small. I felt an odd sense of outdoor disconnectedness, a detachment that has hit me in the face of nature's brilliance before. Has this singular piece of God's handiwork always been here? I wondered. Because I had not been aware of the Chinese Wall's magnificence, because pictures and articles cannot hint at its power, was it somehow less real until the moment that I saw it? And, as in quantum physics, were we changing something so beautiful simply by observing it?

Deer plied the base of the Wall while golden eagles rode thermals along its face. Squirrels raced away from us, staying in the trail like cattle being herded down a narrow road. We made dinner at lunch for a second day running, unwilling to cook on an open fire in the evening. The blonde black bear that joined us for dinner and the noisy deer at midnight had combined to set our nerves on edge. Once I gave a brief start to a movement paralleling me in the trees. The movement stopped when I stopped, as is the habit of shadows.

We walked the length of the wall in hot sun, eventually rounding over Larch Hill. Feathery alpine larch, which covered much of the hillside, is one of only two conifers that shed their needles in the winter. Each fall, a stunning display of golds, yellows, and rusts precede the needle drop. Larch contains a great deal of resin, which makes the rot-resistant wood a favorite for use in wet conditions. Miners, for example, often preferred larch for mine shaft timbers and props.

At the base of Larch Hill, small, glass-calm My Lake felt like a perfect place for a planned rest day. We hung the food from a high limb on one of the lacy larches, then set up camp on the opposite side of the lake.

When we talked of building a fire for cooking, we thought of walking up Larch Hill away from the lake to minimize bear attractants. "What do you want to do?" I asked Kate.

"Eat here, but not get eaten by grizzly bears," came the answer. Kate is so often a cool head, but here she gave me a warm, lingering hug. Every once in a while even her stress level tops out. In the end the lake felt large enough for us to safely cook on the far side, near where we'd hung the food.

A half dozen mule deer quickly took up residence with us and began pawing the earth in search of salt. Rarely did they wander more than 40 yards from the tent. By the middle of our rest day, three of the deer grew particularly bold, lying down in the shade of the trees just adjacent to where Kate and I lay resting in the tent. One, an older fawn, marched up to the tent, then pressed his nose against the mosquito netting to better look in on us. As we had only a week earlier finished reading Marjorie Kinnan Rawlings' *The Yearling*, the fawn quickly became "Flag."

> . . . He left her and slipped into the shed to Flag. There was no time to sit and talk. He let Flag smell his hands and shirt and breeches.
>
> "That's bear smell," he told him. "You run like lightnin' do you ever smell it clost. And that's wolf. Since the flood, they're wusser'n the bear, but we shore cleaned 'em out this mornin'. There's three-four left, and you run from them. . . . You jest run from ever'thing."
>
> Flag switched his white tail and stamped his feet and tossed his head.
>
> "Don't you say 'No' to me. You listen to what I tell you."

We took Flag and his friends' constant nighttime ruckus as a blessing. We reckoned that happy deer surrounding the tent meant a paucity of bears. Still I slept lightly, awakened by the smallest noise or the distant, muffled roar of a jet passing over the Bob. It's an odd dichotomy, this smashing together of modern technologies and caveman sensibilities. Far overhead people flying between meetings in Chicago and Seattle agonized over "Chicken or beef?" There on the ground I wondered about grizzly bears and if one might make a meal of us in the night.

We really do live in two worlds, the physical and the cerebral. Reading aloud to each other at night spirited Kate and me away to different places and times. For a moment the sore muscles and bear thoughts disappeared. Even writing in my journal *about* my fears of a grizzly stalking the tent during a previous night took me away from those fears. For a moment I could forget that I was in that same tent, in the same kind of country, with the same potential boogeymen hiding in the shadows. At home, with cancer knocking on our door, with another doctor's appointment just ahead that could change our world, Kate and I sometimes sought escape in movies. For two hours, we could sink into a story of someone else's making and forget our own nightmare. But when the show ended, the cancer remained. We quit watching movies for a while. The conflict between escapism and reality hurt too much, coming to The End and realizing that nothing had changed.

◪

Kate's six weeks of radiation treatments ended the week before Christmas 1994, a couple of days after my brother, Steve, called from Florida. Steve is a strong Christian. "Man can do lots," he told me, "but God could simply remove the cancer from Kate. We are roughly halfway through our earthly lives, Scott, and I want you to be there in heaven with us. To wait is to risk. I don't want to get to heaven and have God say, 'Why didn't you tell them, Steve?'" Steve said his group would pray on a cloth and send it to Kate to heal her, as they had done for others. It's true that I have not always received my brother's thoughts comfortably. Yet the handkerchief has been at our bedside since the day it arrived in Seattle a week later.

And then, our first major breakthrough. Dr. Cain had already felt shrinkage of the tumor during a physical examination of Kate. A CAT scan halfway through the radiation treatments had similarly revealed a positive response. Just before Christmas Kate underwent a postradiation treatment CAT scan in Corvallis, in preparation for our next appointment in Seattle. On December 26 we stopped at Good Samaritan Hospital on our way out of town. I waited at the emergency turnaround as Kate ran inside to pick up the scans. Back at the car, oblivious to any thought that she should wait for our Seattle doctors, Kate ripped open the envelope that was attached to the CAT scan folder. She read the report quietly and then cried out in joy. I grabbed it out of her hands. The words required no doctor's translation:

> *No visible tumor. Essentially the CAT scan of a normal,*
> *32-year-old female.*

◰

The yearling mule deer that had poked its nose into our tent so bonded to us during our rest day at My Lake that it followed us as we hiked on toward Spotted Bear Pass. At times Flag paralleled us in the trees; other times he followed us directly down the trail, pert and happy, with shining eyes and the wet nose of a giant puppy dog. After 20 minutes Kate turned to the yearling and scolded, "Flag, you're supposed to stay with your party, not with us." Flag looked at Kate inquisitively, then jumped back into line as we walked on. At Spotted Bear Pass, roughly a mile from My Lake, Flag finally stopped at the intersection of the trails, tail and nose twitching, and watched us depart.

We opted to walk down the Spotted Bear River rather than along the CDT proper, which passed Lake Levale, as we had been told the latter route would be crowded. Twelve miles on, having seen no one all day, we stopped to camp in the vicinity of the Pentagon Ranger Station. The following morning our route turned up Pentagon Creek, toward Switchback Pass, climbing initially along a sidehill high above the valley.

Walking along in cold shadows, we approached a blind corner. Without warning, a small cottontail rabbit came bouncing around the curve toward us, oblivious to our presence. Down the trail it hopped, filled with purpose, until with a final jump the rabbit bounced headlong off my shins and fell on its back, dazed. The perplexed rabbit glared up at me, then quickly gathered itself, scampered across my feet, ran to Kate, paused to look up again, sidestepped her, and then kept bouncing down the trail.

My dim mind slowly realized that this odd behavior could best be explained by fear brought on by pursuit. Before I had time to consider what form the pursuer might take, a pine marten came loping around the corner, looking ever so much like Pepe Le Pew, the skunk from the Warner Bros. cartoons. Upon seeing Kate and me, the marten jumped eight feet sideways straight into the trees, then chattered at us gruffly for our interference. We had, inadvertently, saved the rabbit. But what an odd chase, half-speed yet businesslike, as if both had clocked in for the day and expected the hunt to last until the next coffee break.

The trail dipped to Pentagon Creek before crossing the valley and eventually starting up Switchback Pass. I pulled on my sandals to carry Kate across the creek. She didn't want to get her leggings wet and develop blisters as we walked, because with her lymphedema, blisters could cause uncomfortable leg swelling. After using my watch thermometer to check the water's temperature, Kate yelled out that the creek was running at 40 degrees. By the first trip back across for one of the packs, I could no longer feel my feet. The only thing I did feel was extraordinary gratitude that the creek wasn't running waist deep.

Atop Switchback Pass, five miles and 2,600 vertical feet later, we ate lunch. Behind us, the Chinese Wall and Turtlehead and Amphitheatre Mountains textured the landscape. Nearer at hand, massive and rocky Kevan, Table, and Pentagon Mountains stood over the pass like the giant turrets of a magical castle. We sat like kings looking over our empire, content for the moment to realize that though the steep climb to the pass had challenged us, our strength had grown. It had been many days—perhaps a week—since Kate had complained of weakness. In recent days she had often led the way up hills. July 20. Now out on the CDT for over a month, we seemed to be truly hitting our stride.

◢

Back in Seattle, preparing for our checkup with the clear CAT scans in hand, a nurse casually commented that she couldn't believe how thick Kate's file was. The nurse's remark cut deeply. Two years earlier, while saying goodbye to our Portland oncologist after the radical hysterectomy that we hoped had removed Kate's cancer, I had asked if he would be offended if I told him I never wanted to see him again.

"Not at all," he replied. Holding Kate's slim file aloft, he smiled.

"You've got it just right, a nice skinny file. I worry about the people with the big thick ones."

Drs. Koh and Cain shared our happiness about the Christmas CAT scan that showed no visible tumor. They reminded us, however, that the CAT scan slices had a four-millimeter resolution—roughly the thickness of two stacked quarters—and hence could have missed remnant tumor. Regardless, a CAT scan provides gross scale imaging; it is incapable of showing cancer that might remain on a *cellular* basis. Our doctors happily celebrated with us, but then helped us realize that while a clear CAT scan was a necessary step in the process, it did not guarantee that Kate was cancer-free. Dr. Koh went so far as to say he felt the tumor was likely under control. He and Dr. Cain declared themselves most worried at this point about other cancer cells having already departed the tumor area. They also expressed concern that Kate's white blood cell count had still not recovered from the chemotherapy, meaning that her immune system was still depressed. The treatment plan remained fixed: a six-week wait, abdominal surgery to remove any remaining tumor, internal radiation to achieve the final necessary exposure, then rigorous follow-up to monitor cancer occurrence anywhere in the body.

Kate and I left UWMC far less happy than when we arrived, suddenly worrying more about metastasis than the original tumor.

In the six weeks that followed, we traveled back and forth to Seattle for numerous appointments, staying with our friends Rick and Emily on most trips. After the appointments we usually departed quickly for our home in Corvallis, but once we headed east on a road trip to Yakima, Boise, and then to our favorite area of southeastern Oregon. We hiked through winter-wet sagebrush there, and I have a picture of Kate tap-dancing on a gravel road in the middle of nowhere. It's a happy moment, but she looks pasty white, with wisps of hair sticking out from under her cap. Mostly she bundled herself in a heavy down coat against relatively mild temperatures. She had little energy to walk more than a few hundred yards.

During the six weeks we waited for the surgery, we worried continuously that the cancer was growing again, metastasizing, moving with reckless abandon throughout Kate's body. Kate spent much of that waiting time on the couch while I labored in the garage on therapeutic woodworking projects. Once I came in from my work to find Kate crying. It's funny how stupid a question like "What's wrong?" can sound at a time like that. A million things are wrong—fear, weakness, needles, baldness, uncertainty, cancer, metastasis, death. But Kate replied through her tears in an unexpected way, "I don't know how *not* to feel sorry for myself anymore."

Kate's eyes were sunken and red, her body beaten. It was as if in that moment the cancer had won, that death was upon us and that all hope had ceased. I began to cry with her. I could only think that there was no dying, just living and dead; to live without hope, with only overwhelming despair, was to be dead. Maybe the hope we needed just then was not for finding a miracle cure, but simply that life might still hold good things ahead. Living with hope—any kind of hope—was the only way we could survive.

One day I hiked into a wilderness steelhead river and fished for hours in the cold rain. It was supposed to be my escape day, but I fished without enthusiasm and then cried as I walked out through dripping coastal old growth. Back home, Kate told me that all day while I fished she had been making short- and long-term plans: sea kayaking in Baja, moving to Montana. . . . My eyes filled with tears once more and she asked if it was hard for me to talk about long-term plans, plans that she might not be around to help me accomplish.

Then Kate began to weep, saying, "This isn't happening to Pat. She's almost made it five years. All I want to do is make it five years. If I can just make it to 2000!"

This was the saddest thought. Kate was lying on the couch under the blanket, her hat on, and I was so overwhelmed with my love for her that I almost burst. Ten times a day I told her how much I loved her. This time when I asked if she knew how much I loved her, she broke through our tears. Eyes wet but smiling, she held her hands apart like a fisherman, saying, "How much? This much?" Then wider, "This much?"

◪

After a night alone at delicate Dean Lake, Kate and I walked on toward the Trilobite Lakes. The trail wound through a recent burn, though thick, deep grasses covered the ground. The lakes glistened green at the base of solid mountains. Rough maroon cliff bands stood out in grand contrast to distant, emerald forests. Behind us, Pentagon Mountain stood sentinel over the valley.

That evening, near Gooseberry Ranger Station on the Middle Fork of the Flathead, we came upon a private horse packers' camp. The group hailed us cordially, poured us hot cups of coffee, and then invited us to share dinner with them. We happily acceded to the ministrations of these Good Samaritans. When someone suggested that we might like to partake of a solar shower, Kate and I looked skyward in thanks, then made a mad dash for our bandana towels. As we clambered for the shower, Mo, the group's ringleader, and Sheila, his wife, set off with their fly rods, saying that the evening's menu required fish. Shortly I rigged up as well. I soon took a dozen small cutthroats, releasing most and returning with two for Kate and me. Mo and Sheila came back with a creel of 13.

Most outfitted groups we had come upon in the Bob ran with about two horses per person. This private group of five—Mo, Sheila, Mo's brother Ken, plus Ed and Donna from the Sacramento area—required but two pack animals, Ken's mules. Just as Mo had the dinner fire starting to purr, the two cantankerous mules broke away. Even hobbled, the mules tore up the trail. Soon the five similarly shackled horses followed, also with an odd three-legged gait. Mo, Kate, and I stayed at the fire while the other four took off in pursuit. Mo yelled that they'd better hurry because he was about to start cooking fish.

Mo ladled bacon fat all over the trout before flouring them. Then he tossed the fish onto the griddle, a full-size cast iron affair nestled atop a beautiful set of coals. I enjoyed some elk sausage while Mo talked and cooked.

Gravel rattled in Mo's voice. "Moved up here from California seven years ago. Montana is a great place. If I'd known, I'd have come 25 years ago."

Mo pulled a couple of beautifully browned trout off the skillet and then added some more bacon grease. As he floured the next two trout in a plastic bag, Mo looked up and turned to the subject of elk hunting. "Taken six bulls in five years in the Bitterroots. Once had a heavy snow-storm snap a branch and come down on one of the horse's halter ropes. Horse couldn't move all night, but somehow managed not to freeze to death."

Horses and hunting took up most of the conversation until almost an hour later when a clatter far up the trail signaled the search party's return. The fish had long been done, a fact that drew a bit of ire from Mo. He shook his head, mumbling, "My brother's got to discipline those damned mules." Then turning in the direction of the trail, he called out, "Let's go, folks—it's dinnertime." Momentarily the group arrived, some riding bare-back, some on foot leading stock, all red in the face from exertion. Once the animals were tied securely to highlines, we gathered for dinner and a recap of the chase. The fish went fast, but I noticed that Kate and I had lit-tle competition for our offering, a couscous and dried tofu dish.

◪

During the six-week wait between the end of the radiation and the follow-up surgery, Kate spent a lot of time at home on the couch. Our concerns about metastasis became overwhelming. We sat in no-man's-land, hopeful for the best but worrying over the worst. Friends stopped by and we appreciated those visits. Our friend Sang brought us home-made Korean food and then led us in prayer. I attended church often, cer-tainly more than usual, but almost always by myself as Kate felt worn, sleeping 12 hours most nights. Usually I sat in a hidden alcove, praying and crying through entire services.

Kate's hair continued to fall out. She felt little energy. Kate's sister, Kim, came to visit. Kim and Kate took many long walks through the big oaks in the park behind our home. One walked upright and strong, the other bent and weary. I'm not sure what they talked about, but the good-ness flowing from older sister to younger sister was revealed by the smile on Kate's face each time they returned.

For six weeks Kate drank juices and ate a diet that one M.D. claimed boosted the immune system. We visited Kate's folks in central Oregon and Giff and Ellen also came to Corvallis to visit us. Those visits were sometimes difficult, in the way that only mother-daughter interactions can be. I want the best for you. . . . I am an adult and can run my own life. . . . The stress wore on us all. Perhaps Terry Tempest Williams stated it best when she wrote in *Refuge*, "An individual doesn't get cancer, a family does."

Ellen recently summed up some of her feelings during the deep stresses of that time. "A mother is a mother until she becomes the child," Ellen wrote in a letter to me, "and my relationship with Kate was still in the first phase. When I heard about her cancer, my heart broke. I couldn't believe this had happened to my child.

"Thirty-four years before, I had been in and out of the hospital for three months, surviving two major surgeries. This experience taught me to be my own advocate in the medical battle. I learned that the patient has to be aware and assertive enough to demand fair treatment, even when they are seriously ill. Since my philosophy was 'God helps them what helps themselves,' I became determined that my daughter was going to win this battle and I was going to help make it happen."

There was often a mismatch in what Kate wanted to receive—support—and what Ellen wanted to supply—support that included medical direction. Many of the difficulties Kate and Ellen had during this time centered around who was in control of Kate's health care decisions. At times Kate became almost crazed by the loss of her freedom, her privacy, and her sense of self-determination.

"Unfortunately," Ellen went on, "cancer can cause people to react in unpredictable ways. You two seemed to be able to handle this tremendous stress only by closing out the world and focusing on the problem. At the time, I didn't understand this reaction and was extremely frustrated."

It was Ellen who first suggested we contact Dr. Cain in Seattle. "God works miracles in strange ways," Ellen finished her letter to me, "and Dr. Cain, in my opinion, was an important part of our miracle."

There's no warm and fuzzy, feel-good moral to the struggles Kate and Ellen went through. Cancer tears at the fabric of a family. Love is the thread that makes up that fabric, and time is the seamstress that stitches the fabric back together.

◪

Mud bogs, both wet and dry, characterized much of the trail up Strawberry Creek. Heavy horse traffic here had long since destroyed any semblance of a walking path. Cursing the worst spots, Kate and I imagined that CDT hikers coming though in early July must have been continuously knee-deep in slop.

Though the miles in need of service looked daunting, much evidence of recent trail work showed. A U.S. Forest Service trail crew greeted us cordially and explained their work. Across boggy ground, they staked logs in place to hold the trail from spreading. Between the logs they put a tough cloth layer to stabilize the underlying soil. Two members of the crew made regular runs to the riverbed to fill special panniers on their mules with softball-sized rocks. When the crewmen opened the pannier bottoms, the heavy rocks rattled to the ground right at the hooves of the mules. The mules seemed not to mind. A crewman then set each rock in place to raise the trail level and help with drainage. Later, they would use small gravel to make the trail even with the height of the log borders. Section by section the crewmen labored; it was slow yet fruitful work.

Kate and I crossed the Divide at flat Badger Pass, cooked along the trail, then walked the last mile into Beaver Lake. The trail, curling down around the mountain, looked to be a mud pit on wetter days. Stripped logs and abandoned tools showed the labors of a second trail crew. We camped near the lake and enjoyed a peaceful sunset. A mallard left a V in the quiet waters. The lake darkened while shadows pushed the sun higher and higher up the surrounding hills.

Departing Beaver Lake in the morning, we heard the faint reverberations of a guitar. Farther along the trail we heard more gentle strumming, joined by a fine voice singing soulful folk music. Soon we came upon the second trail crew's camp. The musician, with a floppy cowboy hat bent to his head, swayed on the log where he sat. He did not see us. Smoke from the morning fire rose around the man, transforming him into a ghostly silhouette. Shafts of sunlight, sliced by the surrounding pines, cut through the smoke. We paused as our musical specter played on, unaware of his approving audience.

Crossing indeterminate Muskrat Pass, Kate and I discovered the freshest grizzly scat we had ever seen, along with two fresh prints in the mud. Dried scat alone justified a good yell or two. This wet—"It's still warm!"— pile set us off like the Mormon Tabernacle Choir. We opted to head toward the South Fork of the Badger, a wild trail that turned out to be littered with even more piles of bear scat. One pile showed evidence of a bear that would stop at nothing for a sweet treat. The heaped scat contained eight neatly punctured plastic jam containers—the small, square kind with four sharp corners.

Sadly, we also found that a motorcycle had torn and tortured the track all the way up the valley. The deep tread marks reminded us that we no longer walked in federally protected wilderness. Badger–Two Medicine country is the scene of one of Montana's most important wilderness struggles. Some believe that this land holds value only in its oil and gas.* Yet these 115,000 unprotected acres provide a critical wildlife link between Glacier National Park and the Great Bear–Bob Marshall– Scapegoat wilderness complex. The area also serves as a link to the impassive rock reefs standing above the shoreline of the Rocky Mountain Front, plus it holds high cultural value for the Blackfeet Indians, whose reservation abuts it.

The motorcycle-torn trail we followed all the way from the wilderness boundary signaled a relatively new threat—motorized recreation. Here, deep in the wild, someone had driven across the pristine Badger River, then raced up the narrow, windy trail, turning wet corners into mud bogs and cutting donuts on moose tracks.

◤

During those weeks of waiting for the intraoperative radiation surgery, I again spent days researching our treatment options, this time at the UWMC medical library and through information available in Corvallis. At home, Kate and I pored over what I had learned. We sought

---

*In 1997, citing overwhelming citizen opposition, Forest Service supervisor Gloria Flora banned oil and gas exploration along the Rocky Mountain Front for up to 15 years. Lawsuits appealing the decision were quickly filed. By November 2001, the appeals had reached the U.S. Supreme Court. The Supreme Court declined to hear the appeals, so for the time being the Rocky Mountain Front will be protected from oil and gas exploration.

information about immunotherapy and monoclonal antibody treatments from our doctors. Dr. Koh consulted with researchers at the University of Washington to determine if either treatment held possibility for Kate's circumstances. Neither did. We also talked with our doctors about the complications of the planned internal beam radiation treatment, the principal one being potentially painful nerve damage. Complications aside, as the weeks went by Kate and I grew more committed to following the path our doctors had set forth. We asked Drs. Cain and Koh to confirm that their planned treatment was our most aggressive path forward. They did.

When we told Dr. Koh at one of our appointments that we were not working, he seemed surprised, especially that I was taking time off along with Kate. I told him that this is what we were doing right now, not squeezing in getting well from cancer at the end of the workday. Back in Corvallis, my sister Suz reminded me that Kate and I were blessed to have disability compensation so that we were not compelled to work, and also reminded me how much prayer had already helped our cause. I agreed with Suz's thoughts. I recalled the many times my mom had phoned to tell of folks at their church—people who had never met Kate nor in some cases even me—praying for Kate's recovery.

I broke down crying while sitting in the waiting room at Kate's preoperative CAT scan. So many memories flashed through my mind, like hearing our Portland oncology nurse saying, "We consider the hospital a terrible place to die." I was reading Chapter 5 of Bernie Siegel's book *Love, Medicine and Miracles*—the part about acknowledging that we worry—when the wave of emotion hit. I couldn't read between the tears. I *do* worry, I thought, *I worry all the time!* I worried about Kate's headaches and the smallest bump under her chin. Are there lymph nodes under the chin? Is the bump a new tumor? I wondered how Kate could not be worrying continuously, and though she was incredibly strong, I knew that she worried, too.

A couple of nights later I told Kate how I had cried during the CAT scan. She, in turn, recalled how the iodine for the CAT scan had made her queasy, and how that feeling made her suddenly remember the difficulties and pains of surgical treatment. Kate's face looked drawn and exceedingly troubled as she expressed fear about the upcoming intraoperative radiation surgery and about the recovery. Listening to her, for the first time ever I got the distinct sense of Kate's soul standing outside her body, looking in but without complete control of her physical self. Always before I had seen the two as one.

"Everything, every moment is frightening. How can we change that?" I asked her. "How do we cope with all this fear?"

That's when, without bravado, Kate told me that earlier that day she had come to an important realization: *She could deal with whatever happened.* Kate had been taking clandestine bike rides and walks that had apparently helped focus her thinking.

"People with the good attitudes are the ones who always do the best, even right up until almost the end," she explained. "I have to live to enjoy life, to have fun. *I can do this.* Why waste a day worrying whether you have a hundred thousand days left or a hundred? It's harder for you, because afterward there is nothing. I live happy, then maybe have a short bad time, then go to a good place. It's not fair for you; you'll be alone."

To be alone. . . . My mind fogged sometimes, thinking about coming into the house and finding it forever empty, or looking into my rearview mirror while biking and seeing no one following close behind. If I was to be alone, what would I do? How could I keep going? What could I insert in that huge hole of lost happiness? Sometimes I felt like I needed a sanity file, something I could fill with ideas that would keep me occupied if Kate was gone. Woodworking? Fishing? A dog? Everything I thought of seemed so trite.

Tears flowed as these thoughts overwhelmed me. When Kate told me not to cry, the tears simply poured out harder. "Whatever it is," she said, now holding me, "if it happens we only have to live through it once. Let's not live through it now."

In one of our cancer books, we'd read words from women afflicted with cancer describing how their husbands just didn't get it. "*I get it!*" I wanted to scream. "This cancer is threatening to take away my life's breath, and we feel so helpless!"

Kate had read something about spouses having seemingly inappropriate feelings, such as *wanting* their cancer-inflicted spouse to die. As my tears slowed, she asked, "Do you ever wish that? That I would just die?"

I said no, but that I often thought about just wanting everything to be over. I did know that if cancer was to bring death, I wanted it to be fast and painless. That was my morbid prayer. I did not wish for anything other than what I had before. I only longed for Kate to be given back her life.

I continued to quietly sob through all of this morbid discussion, holding Kate's hand, unable to look into her eyes because it all hurt so badly. I bit my lip and said that so much of my happiness was her. Then Kate reminded me of how my uncle Dutch had found new happiness with Kathy after my aunt Nell's death. Kate talked about how I would find someone else if she died and how it would be okay. I wept miserably at this thought, and I said that I could be happy doing what I was doing just then, just holding her hand.

That's when, lying on the floor beside us, Tigger let out a big, unimpressed yawn, crossed her paws, and fixed a steady gaze on us. The drama broken, Kate and I started to laugh. Feline Psychotherapy 101.

◪

I landed a 19-inch, football-shaped cutthroat on my first cast at the confluence of the North and South Forks of the Badger River. After lunch we continued on, along a trail now transformed into a full-fledged OHV motorway. Out of the trees, the sun blared down and we began to drag.

Suddenly Kate tripped and fell hard. She looked up at me and began to sob, "My legs are so swollen I can't walk." Nearby was a stream. We moved there quickly to ice Kate's legs in the cold water.

Placated, we headed on, walking in the shadow of Goat and Running Owl Mountains, eventually to arrive at the empty Badger ranger cabin. Weary of bear concerns, we decided to sit and relax on the cabin's veranda. A short spell of reading Ivan Doig's *English Creek* out loud led to dinner at the nearby picnic table. Not long after that, thunderclouds mounting and rain spitting down, we decided to sleep right on the veranda. As the sky turned purple and distant lightning battered the eastern front, Kate continued to read aloud:

And of course one of the things a person always does a lot of in Montana is watching other people's weather . . . the next time I reconnoitered, rain was pushed off my mental agenda. The cloud was bigger, blacker, and closer. A whole hell of a lot closer. It also was rumbling now like it was the engine of the entire sky. That may sound fancy, but view it from my eyes at the time: a dark block of storm, with pulses of light coming out of it like flame winking from firebox doors. And even as I gawked at it, a jagged rod of lightning stabbed from the cloud to the earth. Pale lightning, nearer white than yellow. . . .

The next day's walk away from the Badger ranger cabin took us out of Badger country and into Two Medicine country. We crossed the South Fork of the Two Medicine River a dozen times along the way before finally climbing out of the valley and heading for Marias Pass. A couple of other hikers pointed us onto the wrong trail; we had wanted to end up at the Marias Pass campground, but instead we ended up at the trailhead a mile down the road. No matter, as we happily ran into Janelle Rieger, the ranger from the Welcome Creek ranger cabin 120 miles earlier. Janelle and her father, a retired ranger himself, were about to embark on a horse packing tour of the Bob.

Recognizing us and then looking at me, Janelle exclaimed, "If I'd have known you were coming, I'd have packed the Double Stuf Oreos a little closer to the top!"

When we told Janelle about Kate's run-in with the blonde black bear, Janelle recounted, "Yeah, that blonde black bear got a lot of radio play for a bunch of days. A couple of outfitters saw it and said it was a grizzly. So did Macon, the backcountry ranger. When they thought it was a marauding griz, boy, they shut down camping in the valley fast. They brought in a team to set up camp and draw the bear in so they could trap it or shoot it. When the bear showed up they realized it was a black bear, just like the first backpackers who ran into it had said."

When we realized that those first backpackers had been us, Janelle reached out to Kate. "I want to shake your hand. You knew better than most of the professionals."

Kate was a bit tough to live with after that as we walked up the railroad tracks toward Marias Pass proper. I told her to go ahead and gloat; she deserved it.

We wanted to finish right at Marias Pass because we had walked from there to Two Medicine back in June. Now we only needed to hike the stretch from Two Medicine to the Going-to-the-Sun Road in order to complete the Canada-to-MacDonald Pass section of our Montana CDT walk. Arriving at Marias Pass proved a great milestone. With more than 300 miles under our belt, we felt like true long-distance hikers for the first time. Plus, we had taken a big step toward accomplishing one of our major goals for the hike—to explore slices of Montana we'd never seen. Most important, we had learned that Kate was capable of concerted daily effort—that in fact she thrived on it. For that revelation we were (and are) profoundly and humbly thankful.

After ten days of hiking from Benchmark, Kate and I both looked forward to a couple of rest days, large quantities of food, and some time not thinking about grizzlies. From my journal, it's clear we were thinking about other things as well. In a game of Hangman, which I appear to have lost, Kate's word was S H O W E R S.

Our interest in the good things of civilization shortened our patience considerably. At Marias Pass we tried hitchhiking for only 15 minutes before deciding to tackle matters more proactively. A convertible—shiny, powder blue, '60s vintage—pulled into the pass rest area, and we pounced. The car's occupants, a couple, sat on the curb drinking icy beers. When I accosted them for the short ride into East Glacier, they consented, the decision tilting favorably our way only after we offered some cash for the ride. Jerry and Jackie, it turned out, were pointed toward a vintage car show in Cut Bank.

Kate and I tossed the packs in the middle, then climbed into the backseat. Up front, a cooler of beer sat on the floor under the radio. Jerry hit the road fast. He told us about the car show, yelling to be heard over the roar of the 80-mile-per-hour wind racing past us. Clouds over the near mountains showed rain and, halfway to East Glacier, the sky opened.

Jackie, dressed in a halter top, shouted to Jerry, "Maybe we ought to put the top up!"

"Naw!" Jerry yelled back. Then, signaling to the violent storm clouds with his beer bottle, he proclaimed, "By the time we get the top up, the rain will have stopped." The rain continued to pound down. Kate and I repositioned our packs protectively in our laps, but our faces and heads soon dripped.

Great streams of water began to run down the road. We careened from one side of our lane to the other, while Jerry tried to duck his head tightly behind the protective safety of the windshield. At the same time he lovingly wiped the dash with a towel, but never once did he set his beer down. He even managed to take a swig or two. And for a reason that will forever remain unexplained, Jerry chose not to exercise his option to turn on the windshield wipers.

"Are you sure you don't want to put the top up?" Jackie asked again, by now looking as bedraggled as a kitten who had fallen in the toilet.

"Naw, hell, it's almost done," Jerry hollered back as the rain stepped up another notch.

The rain actually did stop just as we pulled into East Glacier. Jackie grabbed some towels from the trunk and she and Jerry proceeded to tenderly dry off the car's leather interior. Moments later they tooted the horn, waved, and departed for Cut Bank. Kate and I stood on the sidewalk, watching them depart and pondering a highly perplexing question: After ten days in the backcountry, which comes first, food or a hot shower? Food won out two to zero. We quickly headed into Serrano's for a Mexican meal.

That first meal eaten, I ordered a second.

◢

On the night before the intraoperative radiation treatment (IORT) surgery, February 7, 1995, we asked Dr. Cain for a thorough description of the surgical procedure. She provided one and as always we were glad her plans included checkpoints and contingencies. First, she explained, she would complete a thorough exploration of the body cavity to help determine that the cancer had not spread away from the tumor area in the cervix. If the cancer had spread, she would call off the IORT. Otherwise, she would remove as much of any remaining tumor as possible, then identify the exact area for Dr. Koh's internal radiation exposure. She also reiterated something she and Dr. Koh had been mentioning all along, that they would have radioactive iodine-125 seeds for implantation as a backup treatment should no tumor be visible for IORT exposure. Our Portland oncologist had marked the original site of the tumor with metal clips, thus allowing for I-125 seed placement to best eradicate remnant cancerous cells. Dr. Cain said that after the surgery, we would again consider another round of chemotherapy, though Kate's blood results still did not show sufficient immune system recovery.

We had checked in the night before the surgery so Kate could get pumped up on two blood transfusions and take five sequential enemas. That night Kate would not take any sedatives, remembering a bad experience she'd once had with Valium. I slept fitfully through the night, though Kate slept on. When we woke at 6:15 she went to the bathroom, then said, "If they're not coming until 6:45, I'm going back to sleep." And she did.

I cried as we wheeled Kate to surgery, then sobbed as I let her go. She just waved at me with red, tearful eyes and was gone. Those sunken eyes were not hers; those eyes did not sparkle. When the doors closed I walked to the empty waiting room, sat, stood, then aimlessly wandered downstairs for coffee. Back at the waiting room, a couple of folks arrived and soon started talking jovially. My anguish and face-in-the-hands posture threw a curtain of tension over the room and they soon quieted.

It was still early and I prayed for 20 or 30 minutes, until suddenly I felt a hand on my arm. Joanna Cain, dressed in surgical scrubs, was sitting beside me. "They're having a bit of trouble getting Katie's anesthesia going," she said, "so we won't be starting at 7:45, probably not until past 8:00. She's throwing up a bit, also. I asked how she was doing, and she said fine, but Katie said she didn't think you were doing so well. She thought maybe I should come out and see you."

Tears swelled my eyes thinking about Kate's toughness and incredible selflessness. I stammered, "It's just so much stress."

"I know," Joanna said soothingly. "I've sat in your chair before and it's not easy. Everyone in the operating room knows my routine. I'll have them call out when we get started, and every once in a while thereafter. When we take samples for biopsy, you'll know the results as soon as we do."

Dr. Cain rubbed my back and left. Others around the waiting room glanced at me and talked even more quietly than before. I wrapped the cloth my brother Steve had sent around my hands, and then I wrote a long prayer:

> . . . *Lord, give me strength for Kate to rest against. Help me to be*
> *happy and positive and confident. We must win this battle. Kate is*
> *the wrong person for this disease. . . . Why are you testing us? Why*
> *this pain and loss of innocence? We must believe that you have a*
> *purpose. We must be up to your design, but please help it to end*
> *soon. We have a life to return to. . . .*

A wall phone rang at 8:15. I jumped to answer it while everyone else sat, uncertain whether to respond. "Mr. Bischke? Dr. Cain wants you to know that the surgery has started."

Prayer. Closed eyes. Rolling stomach. Rrrrr-ing. 8:45.

"Mr. Bischke? Dr. Cain wants you to know that it's going slowly because there are lots of adhesions.* But everything is fine."

Giff and Ellen arrived. Ellen hugged me, saying that with new snow the Cascades looked truly beautiful that day.

Rrrrr-ing. 9:45. "Mr. Bischke, Dr. Cain wants me to tell you that everything is progressing as planned, and that she found no new cancer—in fact she could not find the original tumor at all." The compassion of Dr. Cain's phone calls drew me to tears. Here was a woman acting as our agent in health, empowered as Kate's physician but never, never forgetting that it was our future that was being cast.

Soon a page sounded over the loudspeaker, "Dr. Wui-jin Koh to the operating room." Time for intraoperative radiation. But it seemed not long afterward that a tap on the shoulder brought me out of prayer. Wui-jin asked if I wanted to step into the private room next door. He reported that the surgery had gone well, that he and Jim Raymond, his chief resident, had observed some of it, and that Dr. Cain seemed quite pleased.

---

*Trauma such as abdominal surgery can cause tissues to bond to other tissue or organs and form bands of scarlike tissue, or adhesions.

Wui-jin reported that no additional cancer had been found, which I already knew. Additionally, given that no tumor was visible, he had used I-125 implants as planned rather than intraoperative radiation treatment.

Dr. Koh left me alone, smiling. I found two pennies on the floor in front of me and slipped them into my wallet for forever. Dr. Cain arrived not long afterward, repeating that all had gone well. She complimented our Portland doctor for leaving the clips that guided Dr. Koh's placement of the radiation seeds. Twice as she talked, I interrupted to ask, "At this point, is there anything that could have gone in any way differently, that would have made you happier?" Both times she gave the same answer, "As of this moment, everything is as good as we could hope for."

Back upstairs at 6NE, Kate returned from the recovery room, but gained consciousness ever so slowly. I paced the room with restless excitement, anxious for Kate to wake so that I could share the good news. A nurse I had never seen checked on Kate and then, out in the hall, asked me, "How long has your wife been sick, anyway?"

Pondering the question I realized again, as I had months earlier, that Kate had still never really been "sick" at all. True, Kate had suffered from her cancer treatments—swelling legs, surgical recoveries, chemotherapy miseries, radiation-induced digestion woes—but never really from the adenocarcinoma itself. The cancer had been the grizzly outside our tent, full of raw and uncontrollable power, capable of unthinkable evils. And perhaps now we had finally banished the bear. Perhaps.

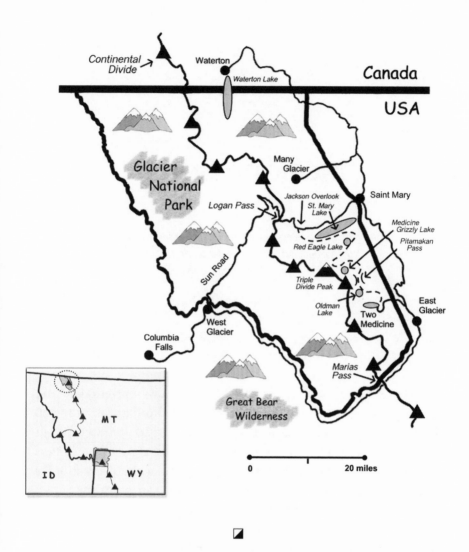

Our hiking route (**Chapter 7**) from Two Medicine in Glacier National Park
north to the Jackson Overlook. Our route is shown as a dashed line.
The inset shows the approximate area included in the larger map.

◪

SEVEN

Medicine Grizzly

I talk when bears are active on brushy trails around blind corners.
Not too loud, but I talk. Sometimes I sing quietly, but
never country and western.

DOUG PEACOCK
Grizzly Years

I T WAS THE END of July 1998. Three rest days separated Kate and me from the date our permit would allow us to start hiking the 40 miles we had remaining in Glacier National Park. We washed our clothes, caught up on correspondence, and spent a great deal of time peacefully reading. Reunited with our car, we drove to the west side of the park, to Columbia Falls and Kalispell, and ate well. We spent one blistering afternoon sitting out the heat in a movie theater and then later in a grocery store freezer section. Music on the car radio and music piped into the grocery store clearly made an imprint on Kate. After seeing me bemusedly watch her toes tap, she explained, "I must be getting used to Montana, country music is actually starting to sound pretty good."

Returning to East Glacier on our last rest day, we drove the Sun Road over Logan Pass. Rather than going to the Logan Pass Visitor Center, we chose to park at the far end of the asphalt, sit alone on the rock wall, and look east toward Going-to-the-Sun Mountain. Jackson Overlook, partway up Going-to-the-Sun Mountain, is where we had stopped hiking south a month earlier. Beginning the next day, Kate and I would hike north from Two Medicine to Jackson Overlook, thereby completing our walk of Montana's CDT north of MacDonald Pass.

For a time we sat quietly alone. Later, shortly after Kate had left for the car, I heard a commotion and looked back. A crowd of tourists led by a park ranger was herding a sturdy mountain goat down the pavement. The goat wove its way through RVs and SUVs, dodged a surprised Kate, then hopped the rock wall an arm's length from where I sat. The ranger arrived, gave me an exasperated look, and exclaimed, "Sometimes I feel like a glorified shepherd." A crowd of excited folks quickly surrounded us, cameras snapping like castanets. For his part the big billy dropped off the hill and then stopped to graze, unconcerned, behind a notice that declared, Area Behind this Sign Closed to Public Entry for Resource Protection.

Wildlife holds an uncanny power over man. Energized parents lifted mesmerized children onto their shoulders to better see over the crowd. Folks spoke with such awe that I felt privileged to observe their reactions. One woman took a picture, then turned to her compatriot and gushed, "I *love* this vacation!"

Driving again later, Kate and I watched the mountainsides for animals and soon came to a short line of cars. People's awe of wildlife sometimes leads them to stupid places. Above us, on a hillside along Saint Mary Lake, a grizzly jogged across the slope. A hundred yards behind, climbing high above the road, a tourist and his camera pursued.

Back in East Glacier, Kate and I hooked up again with Mel, our Jammer-driving friend who had dropped us a month earlier at MacDonald Pass near Helena. She agreed to meet us for breakfast the next morning, drop us at our hike's start at Two Medicine, and then shuttle our car up to the Jackson Overlook.

In East Glacier that night, Kate and I ate our last Mexican food before returning to the trail. I take excessive joy in eating at Mexican restaurants. Strange, because I tend toward rice and beans—just like on the trail—yet there's something about sitting down to Mexican food that I find therapeutic, maybe even a little spiritual. As we ate, rain bounced on the pavement outside Serrano's. Thunder echoed off the mountains.

Suddenly a deafening *"Crr-ack*#!"* resounded at the exact instant a violent white flash exploded in the street. Silence gripped the restaurant.
Lights flickered. Then from the kitchen came the drone of a staticky
radio, spouting the latest news about President Clinton and Monica
Lewinsky.

Bring on the lightning, we thought, bring on the griz; it's time to get
out of the front country.

◨

Like a well-practiced athlete, Kate moved efficiently through the steps of
recovering from the abdominal surgery that included placement of the
radioactive I-125 seeds. Dr. Cain and her residents visited regularly. Dr.
Cain shared our happiness that everything had gone as well as possible,
but she threw some caution into the revelry. Adenocarcinomas are noto-
rious for recurring years later, she told us. Dr. Koh had also mentioned
this fact. Duly noted, Kate and I thought. But for the time being we could
only focus on the positive; we could only pour all our energies into getting home.

For the week of our stay in UWMC, we were again principally cared
for by Jana Ghosn, the head nurse on 6NE. During Kate's week of
chemotherapy three months earlier, Jana had taken us under her wing
and worked hard to make Kate comfortable. Petite and striking, Jana pos-
sessed a solid confidence about her role on the ward. She steered Kate's
care where she had the latitude and demanded care from the physicians
where she did not. We had excellent care from all of the 6NE nurses, but
always felt most comfortable with Jana looking after Kate.

As with each of Kate's hospital stays, I slept every night at her bedside.
When Kate was in need, I went to the nurses' station personally rather
than ringing the buzzer. With Jana especially, I shared what was happening with Kate at that moment or since Jana's last shift. Jana made me feel
that my reports were as important to her as the charts at Kate's bedside.

I often turned to Jana to talk some sense into Kate when Kate hit a
stubborn streak. Pain management proved a continuous rub point with
Kate. One night several days after the surgery, Kate refused any pain medication. Grimacing, she said that if she could stay off the Demerol it

might be a sign that she was getting better. I recruited Jana to explain that pain was not a requirement for healing. Kate responded better to Jana's opinion than mine. After Jana left to get the meds, Kate looked at me and said, "Now I feel wimpy. I would have killed for this little pain on Monday."

As the need for pain management diminished, we prepared to leave. Kate had passed gas, had walked the corridors, had taken a final blood transfusion, and had even eaten a bit. As we made ready to check out, Kate looked over the medications she had been given to take home. Her mood turned acerbic. "*Fifteen* estrogen pills? I'm supposed to take these the rest of my life and they give me *zero* refills!"

Still, Kate's sharp tone couldn't overcome the elation we felt at going home. Maybe, just maybe, the cancer was finally gone. Certainly that thought carried over as news of the positive outcome of the surgery spread. After my sister Suz explained the surgical results to her our nieces, Brittney and Jordan, Suz asked, "Do you know what this means?"

"Yes," Brittney replied, "it means that God is going to make Katie well."

Seagulls and rainbows, two of Kate's talismans in her visualization exercises, showed themselves repeatedly on the drive home: seagulls as we crossed Lake Washington, seagulls flying over I-5, a rainbow in purple clouds over the Cascades, a rainbow on a Hawaii license plate. "How often do you see a Hawaii plate in Oregon?" we thought. "Are the angels playing games with us?"

"Look at the clouds. Why are they so beautiful?"

"Because the sun is shining on them."

Arriving at home in Corvallis, we chuckled at the wilted Halloween pumpkins on the front door step. These were the pumpkins our friends had left for us three and a half months earlier, following Kate's cancer rediscovering surgery. Kate and I slipped back into the house gingerly, almost afraid to believe that we might also now slip back into our old lives. Kate settled happily onto the couch to rest with Tigger the cat, and for the moment I dared to believe.

While I was at our local convenience store shortly after we arrived home, a clerk asked absently, "How are you today?"

Handing over my money, I replied, "Fine . . . no, actually *excellent!*

My wife just returned from the hospital and we think her cancer is cured."

The clerk looked understandably befuddled. "Wow, that's great. Well . . . er . . . I . . . I hope the *rest* of your day goes so well."

"At this point," I said grabbing my bag, "it feels like the rest of my life."

◤

Mel dropped us at Two Medicine Lake in the morning. The name "Two Medicine," used so ubiquitously in this country, derives from a time when two Blackfeet groups showed up at Paradise Lake—several miles south from where we stood—for separate medicine lodge ceremonies. The two groups joined their ceremonies together, hence the name Two Medicine.

Kate and I were headed the other direction, north from Two Medicine Lake. We thanked Mel, then shouldered the packs at the exact spot where we'd left off back in June. Farther on, at the trailhead, a woman crouched next to her young daughter. The woman pointed into the mountains, up the trail that Kate and I were about to take. As we adjusted our packs, the woman told her disappointed child, "No dear, we are *not* going to go up there. That's where bears eat people."

Well good, I thought, I'm *so glad* to be back in grizzly country. Indeed we hardly made it beyond the campground before we spotted sap dripping from fresh wounds on a bear scratch tree. In that instant, we stepped back into the wild.

"Grizzlies are wilderness incarnate," Doug Peacock wrote in his book *Grizzly Years*. And wilderness—wild country untrammeled by man—is something we and the grizzlies have so little of left. "If we are to succeed in saving grizzlies with all their wildness," Peacock goes on, "we will not do it by changing the bears to meet our needs. For the first time in our relatively short history on this planet, we will have to be the ones to bend."

Kate and I sang for the bears as we rounded the face of Rising Wolf Mountain and started up the Dry Fork drainage. The track moved in and out of the trees, sometimes surfacing on open hillsides below bands of rock and scree. We walked comfortably, amazed at the well-maintained trails: stepping-stones across the streams, signs at every corner, a bridge over a dry creek bed. High above, like an angel hovering on a steeple, a mountain goat stood on an exposed cliff face.

Then, "Bear!" I exclaimed.

"Where?"

"Down there, on the valley floor." I pointed. "See him? It looks like a black bear." We watched the bear bounce along the creek bed two hundred yards away. Suddenly the large dirt mound behind my "black bear" stood up and started to walk. "Oh, great—it's a griz! A sow and two cubs."

We slipped behind a pine tree and peered out. Kate whispered, "Sometimes I wish you didn't have such damn good eyes."

While frightened, Kate's voice held a bit of comedy. Though a sow with cubs is potentially the most dangerous grizzly encounter of all, our fear—at least *my* fear—at that moment seemed far less palpable than the night the deer marauded outside our tent. Don't get me wrong—our pulses were rocketing. But as with cancer, somehow an actual grizzly encounter, when concrete and identifiable, is not as horrific as the dark, imagined unknown. Strength exists in facing the enemy, in having the opportunity to make choices to deflect the terror.

Kate and I moved quickly up the path, sliding in behind trees and rocks, planning escape routes up into the cliff bands, watching the grizzlies warily. The three bears moved downstream, unperturbed, and showed no sign of scenting us. After taking a long last pause to watch, Kate and I slipped over a hill.

The sow and her cubs set my senses tingling. Every fiber in me turned outward, listening, touching, seeing, absorbing the world around us. Encounters with grizzlies, like encounters with cancer, sharpen our field of focus, concentrate our energies, and demand our full attention. The moment of encounter is raw and wild. That moment reveals our frailty and exposes the fragility of a world we've long since stopped questioning.

At Oldman Lake, a mile or so from the sow and her cubs, Kate and I set up camp. An early evening rain soon sent us to the tent. Bears and rain— welcome back to Glacier, I thought.

We read until twilight. Because I was back in grizzly country, I slept poorly and looked forward to the coming sunrise. I spent some of my sleepless hours practicing a breathing exercise I learned from a Thich Nhat Hanh tape. Nhat Hanh, a Buddhist monk, is a Nobel Peace Prize nominee, a Zen master, a scholar, and a poet.

Thich Nhat Hanh speaks eloquently of mindfulness and of being fully present for each and every moment. He speaks of conscious breathing as the main tool for bringing oneself to full awareness and control and as a means for releasing the mind's clutter.

"Breathing in I say, 'Yes, yes, yes.' Breathing out I say, 'Thank you, thank you, thank you.'" Over and over, until peace and awareness fill the soul.

And mindful breathing provides a way to recognize and conquer our fears. Inwardly I intoned, "Breathing in, Lord, I recognize my fear of the great bear. Breathing out I say thank you for the opportunity to experience it."

And so I practiced Buddhist breathing and Christian praying, unperturbed by my mixed religion appellations. I prayed that I would have courage and intelligence when we met the bear, prayed that I would be smart enough to get Kate and me through. Kate might have chuckled if she knew about my prayers. Yet Kate had so much to worry about with swollen legs and irritated bowels and shrunken bladder and sapped strength that I thought that this challenge, the bear, must be mine.

Cancer and grizzlies both force us to consider our impermanence; both have the power to rudely rip away our complacency about tomorrow's certainty. Suddenly, living *now* is the only assured option. "That's what's changed since cancer," Kate has often told me. "I no longer assume I'm going to live to a ripe old age."

" . . . Breathing in I say 'Thank you for being alive today.' Breathing out I say 'Help me to appreciate each moment' . . . "

Thich Nhat Hanh writes that we are the sum of our actions, and that this summation is a Western way of defining Karma. Kate and I talked once about this profoundly simple idea. If our essence is made up of that which we do, how we react, and what we undertake, then whom have we *already* shown ourselves to be? And who but ourselves could possibly be responsible for what we've become? Why are we walking 900 miles and why indeed are we now cancer-free? Luck? Exercise? Good eating? Medical knowledge? Openness to prayer?

Yesterday is gone. We can only continue to build on our Karma from today forward.

◪

Late February 1995. Nine days after our happy postsurgery homecoming, Kate was back in the hospital, this time at Good Samaritan in Corvallis. She hadn't kept much food down during the time she rested at home. On the day we admitted her, Kate suffered from excruciating abdominal pain. The emergency room doctor gave her Demerol and pumped her stomach through a nasal tube to remove the terrible pressure in her abdomen. After a few hours of observation, the doctor recommended that Kate be admitted to the hospital.

Being back in the hospital totally dispirited us. Every drop of our souls wanted to cut the ties with the medical community, to be able to stand alone again. Now we were back and dependent and, worst of all, not even sure what was wrong. A blockage? More cancer?

Our stay at Good Samaritan was made even more uncomfortable by a physician partner of Kate's original OB-GYN. This man spoke sharply to us at Kate's hospital bed. We tried to explain to him that we only wanted to get Kate onto IV solutions and stabilized, then take her back to the University of Washington. The man spoke of the possible need for surgery. When we told him we did not consider that an option there in Corvallis, he said, "Well you may just *not have a choice* in the matter."

"I really wanted to be in the hands of the team we trusted at UW," Kate said later. "I was afraid of having to explain to the doctors in Corvallis about my history and what they needed to do. I didn't trust their experience, since they'd never worked with my type of cancer before. We didn't know what to do, either, so how could we direct them?"

The stay wasn't, however, without a bit of comedy. The Good Samaritan personnel didn't quite know what to do with the information we provided them about Kate's recent radiation seed implants. Some nurses refused to care for Kate. Twice they bounced Kate from room to room—once to protect the babies on the obstetrics floor, then to put her into an empty ward. Despite acceptable Geiger counter readings, a radiologist wrote special instructions to the nursing staff about how close they could safely approach Kate. Later, when we told Dr. Cain about all of Good Samaritan's precautions, she chuckled, saying, "For goodness sake, we wouldn't send you away from here as a public health hazard!"

Kate and I only wanted to get back to the University of Washington and the medical team we knew. We waited and hoped for her digestive tract to clear. When Kate did not improve in three days, we made arrangements to depart Corvallis, drive to Seattle, and be admitted to UWMC. We set up a bed for Kate in the back of our Subaru station wagon. A kind nurse at Good Samaritan provided us with towels and toiletries for the drive and said she would pray for our safe journey. After receiving a Demerol injection for pain, Kate crawled in through the rear hatch of the wagon. Giff and Ellen tried to make Kate comfortable, then climbed into their own vehicle and followed closely behind.

Near Tacoma we stopped at the rest area for Kate, who looked frightful with a clamped tube dangling from her nose. While Ellen helped Kate past the staring people and into the restroom, I called UWMC to make sure my earlier requests were being processed: (1) nasogastrointestinal suction and IV immediately available as we come through the door; (2) pain medication prescription already written; (3) direct admit through the emergency room already set up; (4) patient room ready on 6NE; and (5) please let Jana know we're coming.

We pulled into the UWMC emergency entrance without incident. All the necessary preparations had been completed in anticipation of Kate's arrival, and we soon settled into a room on 6NE. The doctors arrived a bit later for evening rounds. Wui-jin Koh and his chief resident Jim Raymond, our radiation oncologists, stopped by first. Concerned that the I-125 seeds were causing Kate's distress, I had graphed and charted the half-life and cumulative dosage of Kate's radioactive implants. Dr. Koh looked at my chart with interest and asked if he could keep a copy. He did not think, however, that the implants were causing Kate's problems. Rather he theorized that delayed trauma from the external beam radiation might be the source of trouble. Dr. Koh guessed that Kate had a partial bowel blockage and expressed concern that the blockage might never open completely. Both doctors strongly favored avoiding further surgery if at all possible.

Dr. Cain had similar thoughts. We should wait, she said, rest the bowel, and hope that it opens up. And wait we did, day after day after day. As the week passed, Kate went through a variety of tests that confirmed the near total occlusion of her small bowel. Dr. Cain grew quickly convinced that Kate's woes were not associated with cancer. Based on Kate's clinical presentation, timing, and diagnostics, Dr. Cain concluded that Kate's current problem was located at the ileum—the connection of the small and large bowels.

Daily we waited for any sign that Kate's bowel was opening—gurgles or noises or gas. Then one day Kate said excitedly, "Scott, come here!"

"What?"

"Something significant is happening here."

"*What is it?*"

"I just farted."

We had a couple more of these uplifting moments, but days went by without Kate's bowels moving sufficiently for her to begin eating. Bored, Kate and I took walks out behind the hospital, her IV pole in tow, to enjoy the waterway. I ate lunch in the hospital cafeteria with our doctors. One day Kate got unhooked and we drove to a knitting store. She had found that knitting helped pass the time.

Kate said, "Being in the hospital steals away a lot of personal freedom. A person can only have that cooperating spirit for so long before they want to rip off all the cords and go outside for a walk and some fresh air."

More mindless days passed without significant improvement. While we waited for something to happen, we had to address one major issue: it had been almost three weeks since the last time Kate had held down any solid food. She looked pale and weak. IVs could keep her hydrated, but she could not receive enough nourishment through the narrow lumen of the needle to keep her healthy. To deliver larger nutritional molecules, Kate needed to have a central catheter placed in her chest. The catheter would allow direct infusion of a fully nutritional solution via the subclavian vein.*

---

* A large vein in the upper chest that lies just below the collarbone.

"I've placed over 200 central catheters," boasted the doctor charged with putting in the line, "and I haven't collapsed one lung yet." Still, he balked when Kate said she wanted me to stay in the small operating room during the procedure. Kate held firm, and I watched as the man pushed and grunted and pushed and grunted until the catheter slipped into place.

Kate's color began to return with the catheter feedings, but after 11 days it became apparent that the hospital stay was otherwise doing little good. Wanting to avoid another surgery, Dr. Cain suggested that Kate go back home and continue to rest and wait and hope for the bowel to open up. If nothing cleared in two weeks, we would consider surgery.

Back in Corvallis, we met with a home health nurse who taught us how to feed Kate through the catheter. She also taught me how to give Kate pain medication shots. For two weeks we lived a withdrawn existence, sometimes going on slow walks around the neighborhood, but mostly with Kate reading or knitting on the couch with Tigger. When pain necessitated it, I gave Kate shots of Demerol. Every night I hooked her up to the small backpack that held her feeding solution and its pump. We programmed the infusion rate and then tried to not tangle up in the tubing as we slept.

My techniques as a nurse may have been suspect, as Kate soon developed a staph infection.* One day she spiked a fever of 103.8 degrees, and we rushed her back to Good Samaritan in Corvallis. By then we had joined up with a local gastroenterologist, Dr. Terrance Hill, who came to see Kate and prescribed antibiotics that thankfully broke the fever.

Kate rested for several days in the hospital and received excellent care. Many on the staff recognized her from our increasingly frequent visits. Several nurses—people whose names we did not even know—said they would pray for us. A hospital administrator even stopped in to apologize for the radiation-scare shuttle treatment Kate had received during her previous stay.

With the fever under control, we went back to see Dr. Cain in Seattle. It had now been over six weeks since Kate's I-125 radiation seed implants

---

*A staph infection is caused by a strain of *Staphylococcus,* a common bacterium found on the skin. Staph infections can occur when a skin site isn't properly prepared prior to an injection and the staphylococci get into the blood.

and over six weeks since she had kept down any solid food. In addition, we had reached Dr. Cain's "two more weeks of rest" milestone.

Kate was in great pain. "My insides hurt a lot," she said later. "I wanted Dr. Cain to do surgery to fix my bowel so that I could move on from all the pain and start healing."

The diagnostics showed zero improvement in the bowel blockage. I was dead set against another surgery. I argued that Kate had already suffered too much, and that more surgery would mean more trauma and pain. But Kate and Drs. Cain and Koh felt otherwise. Dr. Cain suspected that Kate's bowel had collapsed and that the damaged portion needed to be resected (removed) and then the ends reconnected. For a moment Kate and Dr. Cain talked earnestly and I felt outside of an important decision for one of the very few times in our entire cancer experience. Then Kate looked at me with hollow eyes and said, "Something has got to change. I can't go on like this."

Days later, in our pre-operative discussions, Dr. Cain told us, "I have my long-case shoes on. The surgery could take as long as 12 hours, even if everything is okay. I plan to be very slow and thorough." Dr. Cain explained that because of her previous multiple abdominal surgeries, Kate's insides would have lots of adhesions and that those adhesions would slow everything down. Dr. Cain said that while making dinner the previous evening she had been thinking about how to describe the adhesions to us. Looking down into the sink, she realized that the sticky clumps of spaghetti in her hands provided the perfect image.

For some bizarre reason, Kate hummed happily as they wheeled her into the operating room. She looked hopeful, maybe even relieved. She told me not to cry, and I did not. Perhaps we were getting too used to this lifestyle. We seemed to be on a treadmill that would not stop. This was Kate's fifth surgery—her fourth abdominal surgery—since being diagnosed with cervical cancer 27 months earlier. She'd also endured chemotherapy and external beam radiation and internal radiation seed implants, yet *still* the end was not in sight.

◪

Clouds hung low over the Old Man cirque as Kate and I started up

Pitamakan Pass. The pass is named for a Blackfeet woman of the mid-1800s whose talents included making war and horse thievery. In battle, Pitamakan dressed like a man and became known as the Blackfeet Joan of Arc. As a horse thief Pitamakan had few peers. She claimed a willingness to marry any man who could steal more horses in a night than she. Pitamakan reportedly died happy and husbandless.

Though happy and *with* a husband, Kate showed female prowess this day, too, marching up to Pitamakan Pass while I loitered, intent on the multihued wildflowers along the trail. Peaks around the valley appeared and receded as clouds formed and flowed and dissipated with the rising sun. Crossing through steep cliff bands, we arrived at the pass proper, a knife-edged affair that paused only for a breath before dropping 750 feet into Pitamakan Lake. Far below, a deer meandered along the lake's edge, oblivious to its distant observers.

We climbed the short diversion from Pitamakan Pass to Cutbank Pass to peek over into the Nyack Valley. Distant waterfalls dropping to hidden lakes, jagged Mounts Stimson and Pinchot, darkly forested bottomlands, and shining glaciers all blended into a surrealistic scene. Moments later, as we were heading back down to Pitamakan Pass, a lone jogger appeared out of the clouds. We did a double take—*a jogger?* Seven miles in from Two Medicine, the man carried no spare clothing, no bear spray, and no water or food. He wore thin runners' togs. Now here's a guy with a numbing lack of intelligence, I thought. The man told us his loop covered roughly 20 miles, from Two Medicine over Pitamakan and Dawson Passes and back. He warned us of grizzly bears around Atlantic Creek. Thanks and have a fun run, we waved.

The jogger disappeared into a large cloud that dropped just then over the mountainside. We walked on, visibility low, and soon saw movements through the gloom. In another moment a herd of bighorn sheep, eight ewes and five lambs, moved stiff-legged across the trail just 30 yards ahead. The cloud quickly lifted to reveal a band totaling 20 sheep. They climbed up the bare slope above us, seeming relaxed in the now-radiant sun. Several lambs poked at their mother's teats. Others tried to knock each other from the king's stance on a rounded boulder.

As the day wore on, we passed waterfalls, avalanche gulches, and picturesque Morning Star Lake. We camped in packed quarters at the

Atlantic Creek backcountry site, then started out alone the following morning, out of the forest and into the sunshine. Our trail climbed steadily away from the campsite, high up the rocky side of the valley. Soon the blue gemstone of Medicine Grizzly Lake came into view a thousand feet below the trail. Sunshine shimmered off waves on the lake's surface, twinkling like light reflecting off a diamond. Mountains towered over the lake on three sides—mountains pulsating with the rich jade hues of healthy forest and grass. Only a white glacier far up the valley and higher than we stood contrasted with the explosion of green. The glacier trailed a thin white thread down the face of the mountain, a multitiered waterfall rushing to Medicine Grizzly Lake far below.

At least two stories purport to describe the origin of the odd name "Medicine Grizzly." The more compelling of the two goes like this: Calf Robe, a Blackfeet warrior, went south with three compatriots to steal horses from the Shoshones. The Blackfeet were successful, but the Shoshones pursued, eventually overtaking the band and killing Calf Robe's compatriots. Calf Robe escaped, gravely injured. Hiding in the forest (presumably somewhere in this area), he was too weak to even crawl for water. A coyote discovered him and then so did a grizzly bear. Calf Robe prepared for death but instead the grizzly licked Calf Robe's wounds. Together the grizzly and the coyote went out hunting and brought him back life-saving meat. Finally, Calf Robe crawled onto the grizzly's back and was safely carried home. The grizzly was clearly good "medicine."

We paused for a break atop Triple Divide Pass. Here water dripping off the crest of the continent toward either the Pacific or the Atlantic suddenly encounters a third possibility: A raindrop splattering at preciously the right spot on Triple Divide Peak might fragment into pieces bound for the Pacific Northwest, the Gulf of Mexico, *and* Hudson Bay.

Kate and I took the latter route, into the valley of Hudson Bay Creek. The countryside before us to the north and east looked like a book opened to its final pages—one side mountainous, the other side dropping to Red Eagle Lake and then out onto the plains at Saint Mary. The trail soon descended into trees and then heavy brush that we labored to push through. Across the valley, waterfalls plunged dramatically through cliff bands that stair-stepped down the mountainsides.

Soon five young men passed with word that a sow grizzly and two cubs had spooked a couple hiking near Red Eagle Lake, our destination for the night. Although the couple was unhurt, their story had deeply unnerved the young men. The fear in their voices gave us pause. Farther on, while beating through dense brush, I decided to carry my bear spray in hand. I felt like some silly detective stupidly marching into the gangster's hideout. Looking back, I noticed that Kate also had her bear spray drawn. Then, as we approached the area where the grizzlies had been reported, Kate uncharacteristically asked if we could stop and pray, which we did.

We walked into Red Eagle Lake without injury, other than possibly some abused vocal cords. At the lake's inlet, I watched a family as they fished. Their efforts proved successful even though they held their open-faced reels upside down. The mother, who was sitting on shore, reported proudly that the big guy—the one screaming that he had a monster fish on—played basketball on the Stanford team that had reached the Final Four the previous year. When I didn't recognize his name, she said they often called him Mad Dog, a nickname that seemed justified by his current raving. The mother told me they had originally planned to hike up to Triple Divide Pass with their backcountry guide, but then decided to stay and fish. The guide, in turn, had requested the freedom to leave and explore a new valley on his own. I resisted the urge to tell her we had seen their man sleeping behind a rock, about a half mile up the trail!

◤

The surgery to resect and repair Kate's damaged bowel took substantially less than the 12 hours Dr. Cain suggested were possible. Before the surgery started, I walked to a window, unwilling to leave until a seagull, Kate's talisman, flew by. Then I sat with Giff and Ellen and I prayed. Ellen comforted me. Giff continued to be strong in his conviction that everything would be fine; for months he had said he simply couldn't see it turning out any other way.

Dr. Cain called out periodically from the operating room just as she had during the previous surgery. Each time she reported positive progress. Finally Dr. Cain appeared and told us that she had found no new cancer, that she had successfully resected a collapsed piece of Kate's bowel, and that when she'd sewn things back together bowel matter began to flow immediately. I felt a great sense of relief and asked Dr. Cain if I could hug her . . . and then I did.

Kate's recovery from the surgery progressed smoothly, all except for her bowels. She stood, she walked, and we waited for her bowels to move. Morning after morning our team of doctors arrived early, often waking us from sleep. Always they listened to Kate's abdomen and always it stood quiet. During those days of wait, Kate knitted on a sweater. I was working on a sweater-vest myself, though with substantially less proficiency. As the days wore on I challenged our doctors to have Kate discharged before I finished knitting my vest.

After a week it looked as though I might lose that challenge. Although Kate was walking, sometimes at great lengths, her bowels remained quiet. Additionally, pain became a major issue—initially because the pain did not abate and later, more importantly, because Kate began to show signs of morphine addiction. As the doctors moved to wean her from the morphine, Kate became paranoid. Whenever someone entered the room, Kate looked at me with wide, wild eyes and said fearfully, "What are they doing here? What do they want? They're going to unhook me, aren't they? Don't let them hurt me!"

Kate described her point of view: "The 'pain team' came and turned off the morphine machine without warning. I thought they should have reduced my dosage slowly. So with the sudden loss of painkiller, I felt constant anxiety. I couldn't relax. I was clenching every muscle. Just getting through each moment was an effort. I used knitting to pass the endless minutes of those days, but I was forcefully knitting each stitch. Nothing felt natural to me; everything felt forced."

For three or four days the paranoia continued. Dr. Cain, her chief resident John Bogges, and Jana all reassured Kate that everything was all right and that she was experiencing a normal reaction to coming off weeks of narcotic use.

Kate's comedown was not without lighter moments. A few days after the shakes of the detoxification ended, Kate found she had to rip out large portions of her knitting—the sweater looked as though a spider on LSD had created it.

After so many hospital stays already, and with this one heading toward two weeks, we had become fixtures on the 6NE ward. Patients came and went. When I saw their families in the elevator we greeted each other and asked about the day's progress. More than once I heard the nurses quietly inform each other that Mr. So-and-So in room such-and-such had just passed away. Kate and I knew when our doctors and nurses went to a conference or took a day off. We saw the interns late at night, yawning and bleary-eyed.

One of our nurses, Diane, gave Kate a book about knitting and then one day brought by her beautiful dog for me to see. Another nurse, Thomas, brought in his steel guitar to play for Kate. While Thomas strummed and sang some bold blues, Katy Jusenius, Dr. Cain's chief oncology nurse, did a swimming bebop back and forth in the hallway. Thomas's personal and touching gesture made Kate laugh and cry. Later he replied to my thanks by saying, "I was so excited to do it for her."

Sometimes, as I had done regularly during the months we hadn't been working, I left voice mail updates on Kate's treatments for our bosses back in Corvallis. None of our coworkers at Hewlett-Packard ever requested such updates. No one ever requested that we do anything other than pour all our efforts into getting Kate well. But I felt that our workplace, as represented by our bosses, deserved to know a slice of what was happening to us. We trusted their discretion with this information wholly.

Usually I made those calls to work late in the night, past midnight. On the way back to our room I often passed the nurses in the halls. They greeted me kindly, and even those who had never cared for Kate would ask, "How'd she do today?" I continued to sleep in the room at night with Kate and spend all day most every day with her, except when I ran or went to dinner or when Giff and Ellen spelled me.

During one particularly tough day for Kate, Jana stopped me in the hall and said, "You are the most devoted husband I've ever seen on this floor. How are *you* holding up? Can't you take a break sometime?" Jana's words brought me to tears. My own words blubbered out when I tried to explain that Kate didn't get a break, so it hardly seemed right that I should take one.

Kate's withdrawal from morphine coincided with the start-up of her bowels. Slowly things began to move. Our walks became bolder, and we held sufficient rank with the nurses that they would unhook Kate from her IV so that we could step outside into spring. We walked to the canal behind the hospital, feeling the sun beat off the boathouse that we leaned against. Kate drew in deep breaths of warm air and told me how good it felt.

Just short of two weeks after the surgery, Kate met all of Dr. Cain's criteria for being discharged. She was rid of the continuous nausea, eating small bits of food, and showing no more signs of narcotic withdrawal. The interns made arrangements for us to be met by a home health nurse in Corvallis so that we could quickly restart Kate's catheter feedings when we arrived there. We exited the hospital without fanfare, then drove past the Kingdome, where the next night UCLA would beat Arkansas for the men's NCAA basketball title. Kate reclined the seat and laid down but could not get comfortable during the five-hour drive.

When we finally arrived home, Kate walked slowly from the car to the house, physically beaten. As she reached for the door Kate heard a muffled meow, and a silent smile spread across her face.

◪

Kate and I started away from Red Eagle Lake early. This final hike in Glacier Park—to the Jackson Overlook on the Sun Road—would be the longest walk of our journey to date, 16 miles. Steel gray clouds hung low in the sky, though there was little threat of rain. It was a cool day, perfect for hiking.

After crossing the swing bridge over Red Eagle Creek, Kate and I left the main track. The trail immediately turned to a lightly visible tread through grass and wildflowers. The two-mile walk between the drainages of Red Eagle Creek and Saint Mary Lake rambled on through dense brush and wild country. Often we pushed through head-high serviceberry, willows, tall grasses, and overhanging limbs. We soon grew wet in the morning dew. Once we came to an open area on a low ridge. Matted grass revealed where a large animal had slept the previous night. We could find no hair or droppings to indicate moose or elk or bear.

Reaching Saint Mary Lake provided us with a big mental lift, though it did little to improve the trail. The track continued on above the lake, crossing scree slopes and avalanche chutes, then dropping into deep forest and often more chest-high brush. In the open areas, fireweed grew in profusion. We could see and hear cars across the lake, yet we felt detached from the rest of the world.

Kate and I lunched at a creek and then continued on, climbing through lush lichen and moss grottos. A day-hiking family at Virginia Falls signaled that we'd returned to tourist country. Shortly we saw a couple in sandals and knew that road access had to be close at hand (an observation we affectionately know as "The Teva Rule"). Hordes of people soon started coming up the suddenly ten-foot-wide trail. Ironically, after we'd spent the day nervously breaking brush through remote country, it was here that a man rapidly approached us, face flushed, pointing and exclaiming that he and his wife had just seen a grizzly, "Right there, down in the valley, running away across the creek."

After collecting the car, Kate and I had an invigorating swim in Saint Mary Lake and then a dinner stop at our favorite Park Café. Later, at a store nearby, Kate purchased a book about a women's climbing expedition. All the women in the expedition had survived cancer. As Kate tried to read the book's back cover aloud to me, she started to cry. Driving on to East Glacier, Kate became so absorbed in the book that I had to interrupt her before she would look up to see a double rainbow hanging over the Badger–Two Medicine country. Half of the rainbow shimmered in front of the deep purple of an angry storm cloud; the other half sparkled in golden sunshine.

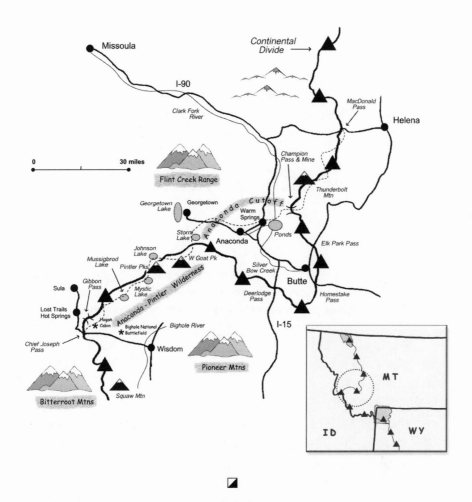

Our hiking route **(Chapters 8 and 9)** from MacDonald Pass near Helena south and west to
Chief Joseph Pass on the western edge of the Pintlers. Our route is shown as a dashed line.
The inset shows the approximate area included in the larger map.

EIGHT

◪

Mental Gymnastics

We were continuously reminded of what we were doing—we could see the form clearly.
There was no way to get the necessary distance, to detach, except to be
outrageous. . . . There was no way to survive except to laugh.

MICHAEL CRICHTON
Travels

EARLY AUGUST 1998. We were back at MacDonald Pass near
Helena. From here on our steps would move us generally south-
ward 500 miles or so along the Continental Divide to Yellowstone
Park. Early in our days of planning the hike, Kate and I had set our expectations to walk north to south *continuously* from the Canadian border to
Yellowstone. Then rough Glacier weather and Kate's leg swelling hit, and
we had jumped to MacDonald Pass to walk north instead.

If nothing else, cancer has taught us to roll with the punches, to be
malleable when necessary, to know when to take charge of a changed situation, and to see the positive aspects that modified expectations can
bring. This change of hiking plans was little different. We could still
achieve our goal, but in a slightly modified manner. Rather than being a
one-directional journey, our hike across Montana along the Divide would
now have three legs. So be it. On the upside, we would now have the benefit of using our car a few more times. And because of the change in
plans, we had hiked through the northern Continental Divide ecosystem

under optimal weather conditions; in fact, we'd only experienced three real rainstorms on the trail in the previous month.

Our run with beautiful weather continued as we started south from MacDonald Pass. Puffy cumulus clouds hovered far to the west, accentuating an achingly blue sky. Kate and I felt giddy, and we practically ran down the trail. We skipped and whistled and yelled and listened for the echoes. Gone were our grizzly worries, swapped now for the concerns of heat and the long distances ahead. Also, we now wore running shoes to help lighten our load and give our feet some rest for the four- or five-day hike down to Anaconda. We had completed a big portion of the journey, 340 miles. Although the numbers didn't quite prove it, we felt as though the second half of the hike was starting.

We gabbed happily, passing through pine forests and out onto tall, golden grass meadows filled with mariposa lilies. Kate spotted an elk, a deer, and once, retreating as she pointed, a skunk. Another time, we came upon the fuzzy ball of a fist-sized baby rabbit. The tiny cotton puff hopped across the track and then tried to hop into the brush for protection. Instead it hit a willow shoot and ricocheted directly back onto the trail, landing wrong side up. When the little comedian finally disappeared, Kate said glumly, "I miss Tigger."

So many times when Kate felt beaten into submission by the medical morass of cancer, our golden furball of a cat, Tigger, brought sanity to her day. Animals can provide a calming, restorative presence at the bleakest times. Tigger had played an integral part in Kate's healing.

"I could be around Tigger when I had a really bad test result," Kate said later, "and she was always just happy. She purred and gave affection and was innocent of the fact that anything was wrong. She helped me through those times." During the endless days at the hospital, we talked often of going home "to see kitty," and soon Tigger began to represent the normality of life away from cancer.

We stopped for the night at a pleasant, if junky, camp between a gravel road and Telegraph Creek. Two withered hot dogs sat on the fire ring, signaling that few animals frequented the camp. It was interesting to realize that in a normal weekend we'd likely never stop in a place like that—at a trashy roadside camp with no spectacular mountain view or trout-filled river. During weekend jaunts people most often seek diamond outdoor experiences. But in the context of a long-distance hike, of tired muscles and thoughts of days ahead and days just past, suddenly the flat tent site, the healthy pines, the relief of shade, and the cool breeze from the small creek provided, quite simply, enough.

Kate and I settled down beside the murmuring creek and read aloud to each other from Stephen Ambrose's bulky *Undaunted Courage*. Talk about a breach of lightweight backpacker's protocol—Ambrose's book weighed one and a half pounds! Mostly we carried thin, lightweight books. We even ripped pages from some of the older books and burned them as we progressed. Yet for this section of the trail, two thoughts overruled our concern about our traveling library's weight. First, we both had a burgeoning interest in Lewis and Clark. Second, after lengthy discussions Kate and I had decided to take the Anaconda Cutoff. Thus, instead of a going from MacDonald Pass to the Pintler Range via Homestake Pass and the Divide proper, we would crisscross the Clark Fork valley from Champion Pass to Anaconda, rejoining the Divide near Storm Lake. The Anaconda Cutoff, favored by all the long-distance hikers we met, eliminates a reportedly sketchy Divide trail segment around Homestake Pass. By taking the cutoff, we'd make our walk across Montana closer to 800 miles rather than 900.

We walked logging roads most of the next day. Much of the terrain we passed through repeated the landscape north of MacDonald Pass— rounded mountains with frequent clear-cuts interrupting the smooth flow of trees. After putting in 11 miles, we considered and then decided against starting up Thunderbolt Mountain. The climb looked too steep to begin tackling late in the day. Plus, as Kate smartly remarked, "Thunderbolt Mountain doesn't sound like the greatest place to camp."

We set up the tent on a piney knoll. Later I walked down to a small stream that ran through the swampy meadow just below us. My rear soon grew wet as I filtered our drinking water supply at the stream's edge. As I pumped, small, cased caddis wandered back and forth along the silty bottom. They busily searched for food, then quickly dove into their carry-along shelters when I dipped my hand into the water.

Watching the caddis, I slid into quiet contemplation. Moments earlier, while resting after setting up camp, I had pulled an unusual gray hair from Kate's head. For so long, I remembered, we didn't know if Kate would be alive long enough for her hair to gray. I recalled looking at the odometer as we drove away from the hospital one day. It read 95,000 miles. I remembered hoping, praying, that Kate would be alive when we hit 100,000.*

◪

April 1995. Now back home from Kate's bowel resection surgery, we settled in for a month of recovery. Kate mostly rested on the couch with Tigger. We went for short walks. Kate took pain pills when she needed them, and each night we hooked Kate up to her feeding pump.

A lot of strange things happened during that month we hovered between medical mayhem and the return to self. We were so engulfed in cancer as a way of life that we could not evade it. Everywhere we turned, cancer reared its head: we shed tears for a friend's mother newly diagnosed with breast cancer; we felt anger over the possible misdiagnosis of Kate's lymphocyst (Why did we accept an over-the-phone opinion from our oncologist? Why didn't we push for a regular appointment or another doctor's opinion?); I sang a Billy Joel song aloud until I hit the line, "Only the good die young," and then fell silent; a friend said, "You must feel like every day is a day you've robbed from death"; a doctor on the radio declared, "No women in America today should die from cervical cancer;" we received a kind phone call from our original, long-left-behind gynecologist; we experienced the rebirth represented by Easter and the flowers of springtime; and we saw so many, many rainbows.

Once at the hardware store, a clerk who recognized me asked how it was that I could be in the store so often, at any time of the day. "Don't you work?" she wanted to know. I explained that I was not working because of Kate's cancer. "Cancer? Really?" the clerk replied. "Is she terminal?"

"No, she's at home and we're hopeful that things have turned for the better," I answered quietly.

But "NO!" is what I wanted to scream. Kate and I have been hit with that question—"Is she terminal?"—a hundred times, and we hate it. We

---

*We've since sold that car, with substantially over 100,000 miles on it!

are all terminal! And "terminal" is such a coldly negative word. "Terminal" leaves no room for possible healing, no room for quality of life issues, no room for future happiness even *within* the context of death, no room for hope.

◤

In the morning we followed a reasonable trail, complete with CDT markers, high up onto Thunderbolt Mountain. There we searched for Trail #119 in vain. Exasperated after 20 minutes of hunting, map reading, and staring at a trail intersection that did not match any information we had, Kate said, "This is one of those times when you know exactly where you are and exactly where you're going, but have no idea how to get there."

Indeed, we simply wanted to drop off the mountain into Thunderbolt Creek, the valley of which showed clearly below us. Sometimes the benefits of finding and staying on the defined trail are outweighed by the time involved in doing so, particularly when the destination is clear. We started down into the valley, bushwhacking through brush and marsh, through open forest and across steep, rocky hill slopes. While neither of us mentioned it, both Kate and I quickly felt remorse over our choice of running shoes for this section of the hike. The running shoes provided no lateral support and little protection against unstable slopes, sharp rocks, roots, and abrupt downward plunges. By the time we reached Thunderbolt Creek, our feet ached.

A mile or two down the creek, the trail suddenly disappeared amid a jumble of fallen trees. After climbing 15 feet up onto the nearest downed tree, we discovered that what had been forest on both sides of the valley now resembled a mass of splintered Pick-Up Sticks dropped in a chaotic heap. The woody mess, the result of a massive blowdown, reached ahead as far as the eye could see. Thunderbolt Creek existed only as an unseen idea in the deepest part of the valley.

We talked about going back to find another route, but then decided to fight our way through the blowdown. We repeatedly climbed through the confused limbs of lodgepole and fir to find a horizontal trunk—sometimes two stories in the air—then tightroped along it before hopping to another trunk. We broke branches and scraped exposed skin. Sometimes the trail appeared in an open space between the fallen trees, but as quickly another tangle of trees blocked it. We climbed and jumped and sweated and grew sticky with tree sap. In the end it took us 90 minutes to travel less than half a mile. The jumble of trees would have stretched farther, but the Forest Service had already come in and cleared the final quarter mile of the blowdown from the trail.*

By the time Kate and I walked into Whitehouse Campground, the temperature had risen to the mid-90s. We pumped cold water from the well, drank heartily, then pushed on for Champion Pass and the start of the Anaconda Cutoff. Our feet ached, yet for some reason we were determined to make Warm Springs by the following night, meaning back-to-back 15-mile walking days. Kate stopped in the road to bandage toes on both her feet. The toes looked swollen and pulpy. My feet throbbed too, but I decided the sight of them might convince me I couldn't continue. As Kate worked on her toes, cars drove by, coming from the direction of Warm Springs, home to the Montana State Hospital for the mentally troubled. The car occupants eyed us queerly. Perhaps Kate and I *were* mentally deranged, pushing on through blistering temperatures, walking on agonizing feet.

Though we were walking along good gravel road, the last miles of the day dragged and dragged. We eventually walked right out of the day's heat. Soon cool shadows slanted over the road. In a deep shade on a hill slope above us, two bull elk rested on the forest fringe. They surveyed us with interest, but did not move.

When our feet could take no more, Kate and I stopped beside trickling Powderhorn Creek on the east side of Champion Pass. We soaked our feet in the creek's icy waters as a large, yellow moon climbed into the sky. Near at hand, coyotes began to yelp. We slept the sleep of the tired, burrowed comfortably into the deep meadow grass.

---

*The Thunderbolt blowdown, which likely occurred the night Kate and I camped in the horrendous storm above Lincoln, became quite a bone of contention. The Beaverhead-Deerlodge National Forest initially saw the 130-acre blowdown as 1.1 million board feet of salvageable lumber. Others, including American Wildlands and the Montana Wilderness Association, believed harvesting the timber would be a violation of federal environmental laws, as well as a terrible intrusion into a currently roadless area. As of this writing, the Forest Service has dropped its plans to plow roads into the area for timber removal.

◤

In the six months after her surgery for recurrent cancer, Kate's weight plummeted. With each bodily transgression—the radiation, the chemo, and follow-up surgeries for I-125 seed implants and bowel resection—she looked more drawn. Kate weighed only 104 pounds, 14 pounds less than normal, by the time she departed the hospital after the bowel resection. Those pounds came off an already slim body. And her weight did not increase even after several weeks of taking in 2,000 liquid calories a day through the central catheter.

Along with making several visits to our doctors in Seattle, we consulted regularly with Terrance Hill, the gastroenterologist in Corvallis. Dr. Hill urged Kate to begin taking in calories by mouth. But when she tried to eat, Kate felt convulsions and pain. She said she was frightened. It had been two months since she had eaten a serious meal. Dr. Hill assured Kate that her bowel was sufficiently healed to handle solid food. He ran tests to show her that she had no intestinal parasites. He asked if she really wanted to eat through a catheter the rest of her life.

And so, with great consternation, Kate ate again—small, soft items. We charted her meager intakes of baby food, chicken broth, and mashed potatoes. And we charted the ugly results. Each time she ate, Kate's insides churned angrily, seemingly fighting against the foodstuffs that had been absent for so long. Kate's system turned acidic, burning her throat and bowels. She often bent over in abdominal pain. We tried 24 digestive medications and supplements during those miserable weeks.

I had my own eating problems during that time as well, in particular a bad allergic reaction to almonds. Kate rushed me to the hospital. Because of our frequent stops in at the Corvallis Clinic and the numerous visits to Good Samaritan Hospital, we had become familiar with many of the workers in our local medical complex. Thus it was no surprise when the woman at the emergency room recognized us and, looking at me, asked, "What's wrong with her tonight?"

"It's not me," Kate replied, stepping forward. Then, with a quirky smile, she pointed my way and said, "It's *him*. Tonight it's him."

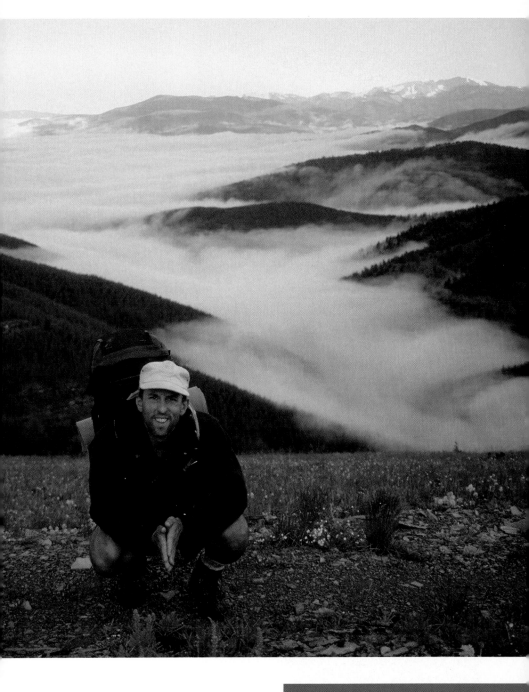

Morning fog above Lincoln, Fourth of July

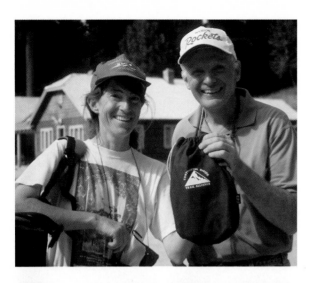

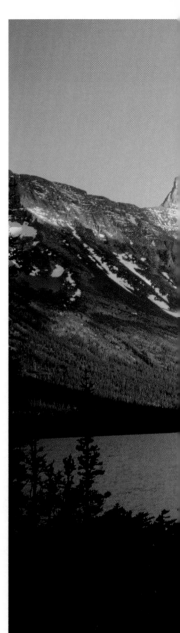

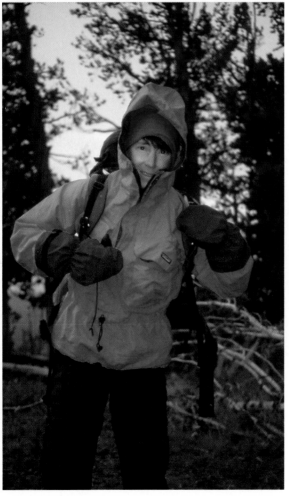

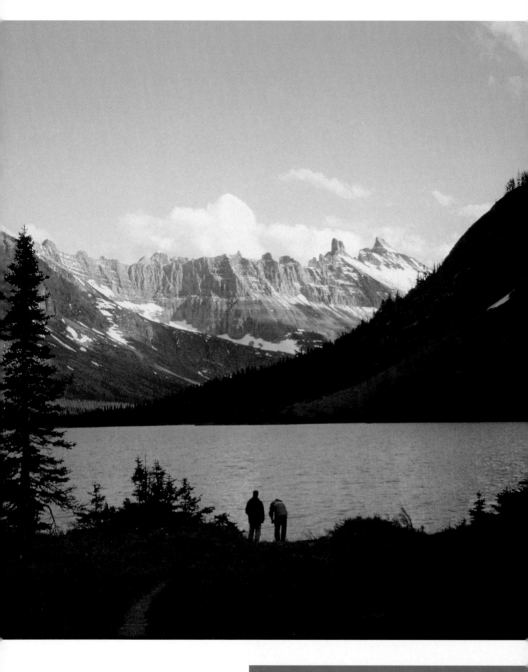

(opposite, top) Katie with Gordon Reese of the CDTA

(opposite, bottom) An icy morning on the edge of the Centennial Mountains

(above) Elizabeth Lake, Glacier National Park

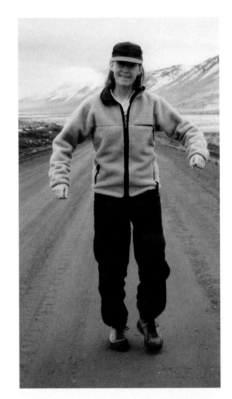

(right) Katie dancing in Oregon's Steens Mountains after chemotherapy

(below) Celebrating the return to Glacier National Park, near Marias Pass

(opposite) Lemhi Pass sunset

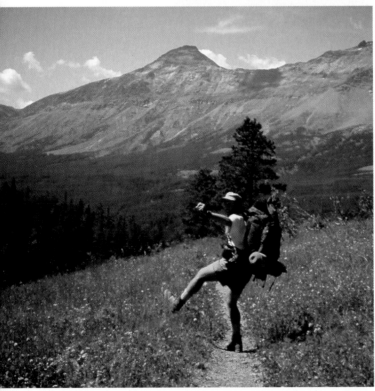

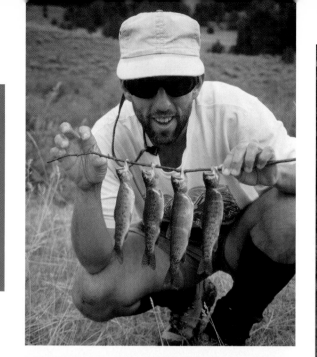

(right) Small cutthroats, but big enough for dinner!

(below) Hiking in Helena National Forest

(opposite) Celebrating hike's end at the border clear-cut, Yellowstone National Park

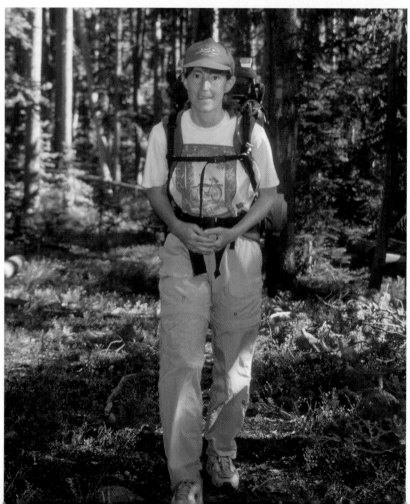

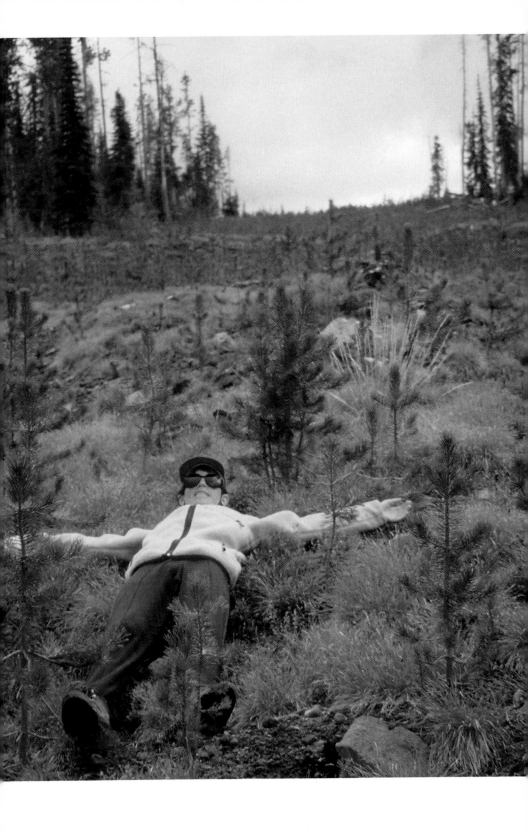

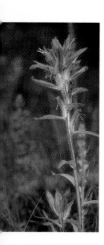

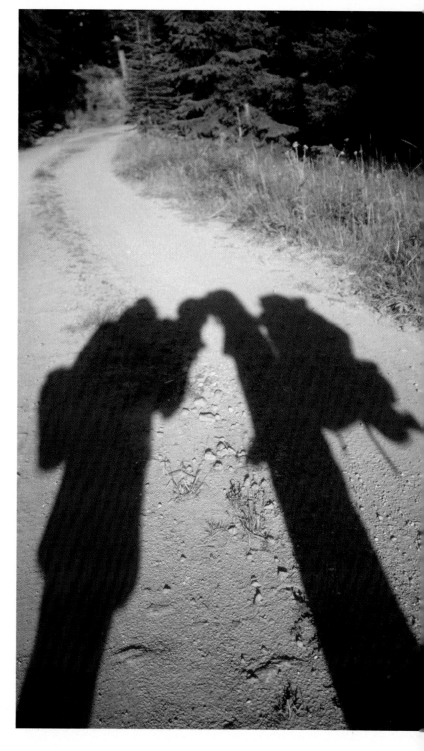

(above) Indian paintbrush

(right) The shadows know....

Kate and I rose early, reviewed the damage to our feet, and stepped back onto the road to Champion Pass at 5:30 A.M. The early start resulted from our desire to beat the day's heat and thus keep Kate's leg swelling down. Though only a hint of light showed in the eastern sky, I worried that we should have set off 30 minutes earlier. The flat plains of the Clark Fork valley promised to be hot and shadeless.

Almost immediately we came upon a herd of elk. The elk browsed on willows while standing, oddly, knee-deep in a swamp. After seeing us in the faint light, several elk snorted before they all headed into the pines. None seemed happy having their last moments of predawn quiet disturbed.

At the Champion Mine a coyote loped past us, just off the road. Here we trespassed knowingly for the first and only time of our walk. Since we wanted to make a beeline for Warm Springs via the Anaconda Cutoff, we hopped a fence and headed straight downhill toward distant I-90. The drop-off saved a couple of miles, which was important to us since we were already looking at a 15-mile day on blistered feet and with temperatures that promised to hit the high 90s.

The Champion Mine area retained the detritus of man's search for mineral wealth. Rusted equipment, tattered sluice boxes, and discarded shaft timbers lay abandoned to time. The mine was started in the late 1800s and soon grew to 800 feet deep, with regular horizontal tunnels. A cage attached by a thick rope to the surface lifted men and ore from the shaft's depths. That ore held wealth; most of the mining district's $350,000 of recovered minerals came from the Champion Mine. Most of those riches came from gold.

As Kate and I made our way through the mine's tailings, the smell of sulfur hung in the air—a sign of low pH and the existence of hydrogen sulfide. Here and throughout the West, freshly exposed sulfides—usually iron pyrites—are oxidized to sulfuric acid via air and water exposure. The acid, in turn, dissolves toxic metals. Left unchecked, these contaminated discharges flow into nearby streams. The burnt orange rivulets emanating from the barren tailings we were passing soon joined cleaner waters and then dropped to beaver ponds. We saw a moose grazing peacefully near the ponds but wondered if this seemingly natural scene hid death on a molecular level.

As part of its Abandoned Mine Reclamation Program, the Montana Department of Environmental Quality (DEQ) has documented 380 priority cleanup sites in the state. Nearly 300 cleanup projects have already been completed. The Champion Mine didn't appear to be one of those remediated sites. Still, the state might understandably claim to have its hands full in this neck of the woods. Just five miles downstream, the tiny creek that we hiked along drops into the Clark Fork River, home to the country's largest Superfund site.

As Kate and I followed the creek toward the Clark Fork, pine forest gave way to aspens. Farther on we found only sagebrush and sunshine. We crossed the rolling expanse of an open hillside, unsure if we were again on private land but sure of our destination—for some time we had been pointing directly at the Warm Springs settlement. Clouds dissipated and the sun began to bake the valley. The day's cross-country travel brought pain to our already heavily blistered feet. Even road gravel hurt through the flimsy soles of our running shoes.

When Kate and I finally reached the Clark Fork valley, the thermometer on my watch read 102 degrees. We walked on, oppressed by the heat, along a straight gravel road devoid of traffic. Once we waited until an irrigation sprinkler soaked us, but its cooling waters quickly evaporated. Mostly Kate walked far ahead. An hour on we splashed our legs with cold Clark Fork River water dropping out of the Warm Spring Ponds. As we had with the sprinkler water, we wondered what interesting cadre of dissolved metals we might be exposing ourselves to.

Since the late 1800s, Butte, home to the Berkeley Pit, has produced over $2 billion worth of silver, gold, and especially copper. Mining operations in Butte have also produced an unenviable environmental legacy—millions of tons of contaminated mine tailings. Much of this waste has found its way into small Silver Bow Creek, and from there it has flowed roughly 20 miles downstream into a series of "settling" basins—the Warm Springs Ponds—which were constructed in 1911 to capture sediments and metals. Over time the ponds were enlarged and, in the late '60s, chemical treatment was added to more efficiently capture dissolved metals.* The Montana DEQ expects that cleaning up Silver Bow Creek will require ongoing treatment. In the meantime the ponds themselves, while providing a bustling wetland complete with waterfowl, songbirds, and trout, continue to collect contaminated sediments—19 million cubic yards and counting. And the Clark Fork Coalition, an environmental group, reports that metal discharges from the ponds still frequently exceed water quality standards.

Kate and I walked around the lower end of the ponds, under I-90, and then into Warm Springs. The "town" of Warm Springs is really little more than a combination gas station/convenience store/bar, a few houses, and the Montana State Hospital. The hospital provides inpatient psychiatric care for adults with serious mental illnesses.

Inside the convenience store, a woman named Sandy Gray greeted us with a kind smile. "More hikers? I've seen quite a few of you this year." Sandy reported that Nick, David, and Andrew (who we met the night we camped in the Valley of the Moon) had already stopped through.

Kate and I bought the biggest cold drinks we could find, then moved outside to the shade of one of the giant cottonwoods lining the hospital drive. I pulled off my socks to find that two marble-sized blisters had grown on the top of my second toes. Kate's toes looked like raw hamburger.

Sitting amid this gore, we realized that with a hitch to Anaconda, we could rent a car and return to MacDonald Pass for our car and, more importantly, our hiking boots. A quick check with Sandy put an end to our need to hitchhike. Sandy identified Bob, sitting just then in the bar, as our ride.

Bob was a young guy, slim and strong, wearing jeans and a T-shirt. His lip, purple and puffy, fell unnaturally away from his mouth. Bob came out of the bar, Budweiser in hand, and pointed to his beat-up Wagoneer. As I carried the packs over to the Wagoneer, he gave the tailgate a good wallop. The cracked window dropped a notch. He grabbed the top of the glass. With practiced ease and only two cuss words, Bob shoved the

---

*Lime addition raises the pH in the pond, causing metals to precipitate out of the water column and fall to the bottom of the ponds as sludge.

window down into the tailgate, then looked at me with a self-satisfied smile. We tossed the packs in on top of empty beer cans and a rusted jack.

Bob climbed in behind the wheel, settled his beer between his legs, and then gunned the motor. We headed out onto the road. A moment later Bob ducked when a cop drove by. "I'm wanted in Butte, aiding and abetting a minor," he explained. "Thing is, I'da never got picked up for speeding to begin with—60 down Main Street—if my eyes weren't so swelled up from that bar fight. I'da seen that cop. Anyway, I jumped bail so they're lookin' for me. Shit, where am I gonna git money for bail?"

Kate and I exchanged a glance as the speedometer crept uncomfortably toward 80. We careened around a corner as Bob took a swallow of his beer. "Have you lived here all your life?" I asked affably.

"Naw, left to go to into the military. Did damn well, too. Later, though, I came back . . . dishonorable discharge."

The smelter stack at Anaconda grew prominent as Bob recounted a recent win at the lottery. "I took that hundred bucks and spent 50 of it on beer and the rest on lottery tickets and shit'n got nothin'!"

We turned toward town and soon passed a used car dealership. "See that Mustang, the hot one with the glass packs there?" He pointed with his Budweiser bottle. "I used to own that thing before it got repossessed."

Bob dropped us at a local auto dealership that also rented cars. He had once worked at the dealership, he reported, but had been fired. Bob gratefully accepted the $5 bill we offered for gas, wished us well, and suggested we tell the car dealership that he had sent us. A genuinely nice guy, we thought, but we decided against his recommendation, thinking we might be better received on our own merit.

◪

The importance of friendship in cancer recovery cannot be overstated. Friends provide cancer patients a stage on which they can once again act out their normal lives. But friends are in an unenviable position: Every bit of their soul agonizes for you, yet they often don't know how to make contact. Rarely do we call someone to chat and ask, "How ya doing?" without something else in mind, maybe a movie or plans for the weekend. For someone with cancer, "How ya doing? I'm worried about you," is exactly the call a friend wants to make. But it's difficult. Everyone knows, or suspects they know, how you're doing—terrible, you've got cancer for heaven's sakes. So "How ya doing?" sounds like a hollow question. And friends also worry that their own health, their own continuation of normal life, will somehow sadden or anger you.

Many of our friends, thankfully, showed little discomfort in bringing us back into their lives. They called or stopped by. We gladly received them and they showed understanding if Kate was too tired for visitors. Friends reached out to us across the gap between the grim world of the hospital and the reality of life waiting beyond cancer.

Sometimes an icebreaker helps. That's where gifts and flowers and food ease the awkwardness of getting reacquainted. After Kate's original hysterectomy, our friends Dave and Pam organized meals for us for a week, meals that came from good people who did not know us yet said they'd also pray for Kate. After other surgeries Jeff and Theresa stopped by with bags of groceries and cooked for us. Linda and Jeff had us over for dinner, as did Randy and Kelly. Doug made us a torte. And the list of kindnesses goes on.

Rachel Kirby spawned one of the most important forums Kate needed for beginning to reclaim her sense of self. Rachel, an art teacher, declared a desire to learn to knit. In Kate she found a willing teacher. Quickly Julie and Colleen joined the group and Wednesday afternoons became a happy, eagerly anticipated time at our house. Early on Kate could do little more than sit tiredly on the couch as the others knitted. She shared horror stories about surgery and chemotherapy and catheter feedings. Kate's friends listened and they cared. Then the knitters shared stories about what was happening in their lives, helping Kate turn outward. Most important, the four of them laughed together in those special moments they were creating. In time, a husbands' running group splintered off and then dinners began to follow the knitting.

Curiously, as the group advanced its knitting skills, less and less knitting got done. Soon the knitting projects stayed in the bag, and then later the knitting was often left at home. The women complained that they always made mistakes during the laughter of the get-togethers. Over time the knitters migrated to another day and eventually to another house. Through it all, Kate gained strength from the group.

◪

Though we had not planned a rest day, my blistered feet screamed at the thought of continuing on the next day from Warm Springs. Instead, we used the car to shuttle food to Bannock Pass and Monida Pass for the weeks ahead. All that, which fits nicely into a single sentence, barely fit into a full day of driving.

Heading up I-15 from Monida at day's end, we stopped into Lima for a meal at Jan's Cafe, just off the interstate. Jan had flowing blonde hair and a personality that lit up the restaurant. She poured us strong coffee and asked what we were up to. An older, sunburned cowboy heard our Continental Divide banter and turned from the counter to talk. He wore a pearl-buttoned shirt and a creased straw hat that matched the deep wrinkles in his weathered face. Clearly the type not likely to be inter-rupted, the man quickly wove a long tale of hiker-hungry grizzly bears all along the Divide between Lemhi Pass and Monida Pass.

"While back I saw claw marks *12 feet* up on a tree near Bannock Pass," he said, eyes dancing as he tilted his hat back. Folks at other tables were by now following his stories, too. "Hell, jus' last week I was cuttin' wood up there and one came a pissin' and a moanin' and snortin' through the brush. I ran for my gun and sent the grandkid into the pickup and— What? Did I see it? Naw, but man, I can tell you that was one mighty big griz."

Once the griz finished fighting over our carcasses, the old codger assured us, the bountiful cougars and wolves would quickly clean up whatever remained. "That'd be shame, too, 'specially if you miss the sheep. I saw a bighorn up there a couple o' weeks back that had a full triple curl."

The tales piled atop one another like logs on a stack of firewood. "Wow!" "Really?" Kate and I exclaimed. We did nothing to challenge his yarns.* Behind the counter, Don, Jan's partner, rolled his eyes a couple of times in amusement.

---

*A documented sighting of a grizzly anywhere along the Montana–Idaho border west of I-15 would be big news. The last verified death of a grizzly in the Bitterroots was in 1932. In the late '90s the Missoula-based Alliance for the Wild Rockies sponsored the "Great Grizzly Search" in

Late that night Kate and I arrived back at Warm Springs and set up the tent behind Sandy and her partner Art's place. In a full day by car we had driven a circuitous route from Warm Springs to Lemhi, Bannock, and Monida Passes, and then back. The one-way trip—320 trail miles to Monida Pass—would take us 31 days on foot.

We rose early the following morning and at 6 A.M., we hit the trail (well, okay, so the Anaconda Cutoff follows a paved road between Warm Springs and Anaconda). To complete the Anaconda Cutoff we planned on two day hikes, one from Warm Springs to Anaconda and the other from Anaconda to the Storm Lake turnoff. Since both the car and hitch-hiking were available to us, we reckoned that not carrying the packs for a couple of days would help our blistered feet heal.

We made an early start, again in an effort to beat the heat and thus keep Kate's leg swelling down. Still, Kate wore a heavy shirt to fight off the morning cold. She tucked each hand into the opposite sleeve, a move that produced a decidedly straitjacketed look.

With no sign of movement at the gas station or at Sandy and Art's home, we set off, immediately crossing in front of the Montana State Hospital. Five minutes down the road a security car passed, its occupants' heads turning as they surveyed us. A moment later the two security guards made an abrupt U-turn, their light bar flashing. They pulled off the road directly into our path.

"'Scuse me," the driver said after rolling down the window. "Wonder if you might explain to us what you're doing out here." Both men appeared bedraggled, with puffy, red eyes. They looked like they were coming off an all-night shift.

I took off my dark glasses, which I had put on in preparation for the day's sun. "We're backpackers, hiking the Continental Divide from Canada to Yellowstone Park," I said. As I spoke, I noticed the men

---

hopes of finding grizzlies anywhere in Montana's Bitterroot Range, as well as several other areas in Idaho. The impetus for the search centered on the Endangered Species Act (ESA). If grizzlies had been found to already exist, the ESA would have kicked in and provided the grizzlies enhanced protection (e.g., habitat maintenance). Credible evidence of grizzlies was not found to exist. As a result, in November 2000 the federal government announced plans to reintroduce grizzlies to the Bitterroots, beginning in 2002. In June 2001, the Bush administration took steps to rescind that decision.

scrutinizing Kate. "It's about 900 miles—Canada to Yellowstone, I mean. I mean . . . well . . . I know this isn't *exactly* the Continental Divide, it's over there, but see, we're cutting across this section and . . . " The guard nearest me grunted disapprovingly, still looking at Kate. For her part, Kate stood back, hat pulled low, sunglasses hiding her eyes, arms tucked in her straitjacket.

The driver turned his eyes back to me for a moment. "Nine hundred miles. Hmm, really?" As I started to stammer something else he interrupted, saying, "We had a report of someone walking away from the hospital. If you're backpacking, where're your backpacks, anyway?"

"Well, you see we're not *exactly* 'backpacking' today. I mean, you see . . . well . . . our backpacks are in the . . . er . . . car back there at the gas station. We're just walking to Anaconda today."

Now the other guard gave an irritated grunt. As he and the driver shared a dubious glance, I tried another tack. "Sandy and Art back at the gas station let us camp behind their place last night and—"

"You know Sandy and Art?" This time it was the one in the passenger seat asking.

"Well yeah, sure. Sure, *of course* we know Sandy and Art." That seemed to solve the problem, and a moment later they drove off, probably headed for some hot coffee or an early morning sleep.

Walking on as the security car disappeared back up the hospital drive, Kate giggled, "You certainly handled that well."

"What do you mean?" I replied contemptuously. "Did you notice how they only talked with me 'cause I was the only sane-looking person in our party? Without me, they might have carted you in for a frontal lobotomy. What about that, huh?"

"Funny, incredibly funny."

◪

A major event occurred during our first frightening steps away from the protection of our home. We had traveled to the coast to stay with our friends Cam and Terri at their family's cabin in the woods. Kate felt wobbly and unsure of herself. I suspect Cam and Terri felt a bit uneasy about Kate's health, but their kind invitation to visit allowed us to take another important step toward normality. Then, sometime in the middle of the night, Kate's central catheter line pulled out of her chest. We woke to this startling fact and decided to head home immediately.

In Corvallis, Dr. Hill reacted to the news impassively. "What this means," he told Kate, "is that now you must really start eating again."

Kate still weighed 104 pounds. Though she had tried small samplings of food, she still relied on the catheter feedings to sustain her. Kate looked ill at just the thought of consuming enough to support herself. Still, Dr. Hill and Kate agreed on one thing: Neither of them wanted her to suffer through the reinsertion of another catheter.

"If you get down to 100 pounds," he went on to tell her, "we're going to have to start feeding you through a stomach tube down your throat."

◪

Having survived our brush with the state mental hospital guards, Kate and I marched on to Anaconda. The Pintler Range aside, the most remarkable feature on the landscape ahead was the Washoe Works Smokestack. According to the locals, at 585 feet tall, it is the tallest smokestack in the world. The stack played an integral, if late, part in Marcus Daly's plan to build a smelting empire based on copper from the nearby Berkeley Pit at Butte. Nearness to Butte, plus ready water emanating from the Pintler Range—smelting used as much as 64 million gallons of water per day—made Anaconda the prime location to site the smelter.

The Anaconda Smelting Company, once home to a work force of around 2,000, is today no more. The smokestack looming over us stood cold, a victim of the declining copper market of the early 1980s. The hotspots left today are all environmentally related. Slag heaps, defiled soils, and contaminated waterways define Anaconda the way smog defines Los Angeles. Warm Springs Creek, which Kate and I were following into Anaconda, is on the EPA's "impaired" water list. Yet even in the midst of this environmental turmoil, mankind moves forward. Farther upstream, along the north edge of town, Warm Springs Creek flows through a championship golf course built on and around some of Anaconda's smelting wastes. The Old Works Golf Course, designed by none other than Jack Nicklaus, is part of a $20 million remediation effort planned by Arco, the current owner of the area. Rather than removing and cleaning the contaminated landscape, Arco and the EPA chose to stabilize the soils in place and then turn the unsavory Superfund site into a golfers' mecca. "Feature your faults," I can hear some clever marketeer saying. Today golfers walk along fairways grown over limestone-capped arsenic soils, maneuver carts around old smelter remnants, and hit wedges from black slag sand traps.

Kate and I walked on pavement to just past the turn into the Old Works Course, then reversed our route to hitchhike back to our car. Soon we caught a ride from a worker at the state mental hospital. From Warm Springs we drove to nearby Georgetown Lake to seek refuge from the heat.

Early the next day, around 7 A.M., we were on the road again for the walk from the Storm Lake turnoff—near Georgetown Lake and close to where we would pick up the Divide proper again—to Anaconda. We hoped to beat the heat of the day, but by damn that morning was cold! And it was just early August. We'll clearly freeze in September, I thought. Walking on asphalt again and again without packs, we averaged 18 minutes per mile and spotted four red foxes on the way to Anaconda. Kate walked jubilantly as it warmed, one part greyhound, one part disco dancer.

My parents, who live in Billings, met us in Anaconda. We had planned a couple of rest days with them at nearby Georgetown Lake. They arrived on schedule, with a big surprise—Tigger the cat! An enjoyable couple of days ensued, including a visit with lifelong family friends, Bob and Nancy Vandel.

One evening at Georgetown Lake, 10,000 six-inch hatchery fish battered the surface with reckless abandon. I tossed a fly while Dad helped Mom recall how to cast a lure. Most of her casts ended up at her feet or in the nearby bushes. Still, Mom showed everyone up by catching a 14-inch trout—as Kate was to later say, "On her first waterborne cast!"

◪

With the central catheter gone, Kate was forced to eat. And in a process that continues to this day, by trial and painful error Kate slowly started to weed through the food items that made her sick. First and principal among those was anything containing the milk sugar lactose. Radiation exposure had destroyed the ability of Kate's small bowel to create lact*ase*, the key enzyme in breaking down lact*ose*. Without lactase, lactose passes to Kate's large bowel, where bacteria ferment the sugar into agonizing gas. Lactase-replacement pills, she quickly discovered, helped little.

Other digestion problems became apparent when Kate ate calorie-dense foods, greasy fare, and meats. Weeks passed when Kate seemed to be in abdominal pain after every meal. But day by day we learned. Dr. Hill provided Kate with a gamut of pharmaceutical and practical tools to fight her acidic system, excess gas, and malabsorption. Kate's job was to apply those tools to best optimize her new digestive tract. Additionally, our friend and herbalist Susan Buhler recommended several natural supplements to help Kate with her digestion woes. Dr. Hill had no issue with the supplements and in the end one of them, powdered psyllium seeds, became a mainstay in Kate's fight to regain control of her digestion. After several weeks Kate's weight started climb, pound by ever so slow pound.

In May and June we flew to Montana and Colorado to visit my folks and Kate's brother and sister. Our families' love bolstered us. In Billings my mom and I talked late into the night, as we've done often through the years. Her actual words were less important than the message of unconditional love they carried for both Kate and me. And by strengthening me, she helped me be better for Kate.

In Colorado we visited old friends from when we had lived there eight years earlier. Still under 110 pounds at the time, Kate looked breakable. Her normally flowing hair grew curly and tight to the head, a reminder of the chemotherapy six months earlier. Our meetings with friends felt like reintroductions. Many of them knew only that Kate had cancer and probably weren't sure if they would ever see her again. I think talking to Kate in person set a lot of folks' minds at ease.

"How long do you guys have to keep worrying about this stuff, anyway?" someone asked. It was probably hard for people to see past our happy conversations to the fact that every single day we struggled; every moment we fought to overcome the fear that Kate's cancer might not really be gone.

NINE

◤

Finding the Lost Trail

This is the animal Linnaeus called Canis lupus *in 1758 . . . his numbers have dwindled
and his range has shrunk, and as is the case with so many things, deep
appreciation and a sense of loss have arrived simultaneously.*

BARRY LOPEZ
Of Wolves and Men

S HORTLY AFTER RETURNING from Colorado, we tackled our
first real outdoor experience since the recurrence of Kate's cancer
eight months earlier. Our friends Jeff and Linda invited us on a
four-day float trip down Oregon's Deschutes River. Their offer was a mon-
umental act of friendship. It had been almost exactly two months since
Kate's bowel resection surgery. None of us knew if Kate could live away
from medical care for four days. On the river, we would for the most part
be out of reach of cars or phones. Yet Jeff and Linda knew how much
being out meant being alive for Kate and me. Jeff, Linda, and Kim, another friend, risked their trip for us. They discreetly worked out the logis-
tics of rushing down the river should Kate become ill; they suffered
through my tears when Kate had an agonizing bowel problem; and they
shortened the trip's final day so we could get Kate home sooner. Yet Kate
and I floated and fished the river—almost like normal—thanks to the
open hearts of these three kind friends.

That trip down the Deschutes started our summer of recovery. For
much of three months we traveled the backcountry alone by boat, as Kate

did not have the strength to bike or backpack. During a visit to Kate's relatives in Wisconsin and friends in Minnesota, we spent several days canoeing down the wild and scenic Namekagon and St. Croix Rivers. I have a pitiful photo of Kate in the canoe on that trip, proudly flexing her arm muscle. The arm—all shoulder and elbow and bone—sticks unimpressively out of her tank top.

On that same journey we heard a commotion 50 yards downstream. Suddenly a large black bear chased a bleating fawn out into the Namekagon, dunked it under, then came up with the flailing little body by the nape of the neck. A frantic whitetail doe kicked at the bear as it emerged from the water, but without effect. By the time the bear and the fawn disappeared back off the river, we had floated directly parallel to them. The fawn's death squeals sounded in tandem with the horrible crunch of bones.

"No, no, no! Make it stop!" Kate cried. A wet, raspy moan sounded from the fawn, then a short pause, then more squeals, feebler than before. "Just die . . . please, just die!" We floated on, silent except for Kate's sobs, far down the river.

We took many more trips that summer, most of them a week in length and almost all in British Columbia: canoeing near Powell River, on the Kispiox, and on a river in the far north; sea kayaking off Vancouver Island, in Desolation Sound, and in the Queen Charlotte Islands. The trips fortified us. Risky? Yes. But it was not in Kate's makeup to sit at home between doctor's appointments. She wanted to be alive again. Those journeys were her expression of life.

Every journey we took into unknown country revitalized our souls. Our minds reopened to the possibility of life beyond cancer. Once, while we were sitting on a wild river, I asked Kate if she wanted me to get her book. Kate responded, "No, I don't want to read. I just want to watch. I don't want to miss anything." Reopening our minds to life also recreated a space for humor. Once, after an icy rainstorm that drove us to set the tent up at midday, Kate's teeth chattered ferociously. "I don't know why we're so worried about cancer," she deadpanned, "when the cold is going to kill us today."

* * *

We visited our doctors regularly throughout our summer of recovery. Early on, after Kate's eating picked up, Dr. Hill in Corvallis dismissed himself. "I'm happy to continue seeing you every week," he told Kate, "but all I'm doing is telling you look better and better. You don't need me to tell you that."

Our travels to British Columbia usually started and ended with an appointment to see Drs. Cain and Koh in Seattle. Always the visits included physical exams, and sometimes they included a chest x-ray or a CAT scan. Once Kate underwent a bladder scoping procedure because of our doctors' fear that something might be blocking her ureters. That fear turned out to be unfounded.

In the backcountry we were able let our guard down. Everything felt so normal. Then just 24 hours after stepping out of the kayak, we would be standing in the hospital hearing hallway conversations about chemotherapy and radiation, and suddenly disaster seemed to loom just one step away again. We agonized as each appointment approached, then waited anxiously for the exam and test results. For months we stood precariously at cliff's edge, feeling as though the smallest imbalance might send us plunging back into cancer's abyss. Yet always the assessments came back positive. And then we would flee the hospital again, holding fast to our next short lease on life, driving hard to get out of Seattle and away from sickness, seeking desperately to escape back into summer.

◢

Kate and I rounded out the Anaconda Cutoff by walking eight miles up the gravel road from the highway to Storm Lake. My folks had hugged us goodbye at the drop-off, tucked Tigger into her cat carrier, and left to drop our car at Monida Pass, 306 trail miles to the south, before heading home to Billings.

The packs, heavy with nine days of food, pulled hard on us. Still, when the trail crossed through the first field of wildflowers just past Storm Lake, I breathed deeply and felt the return of backcountry peace. The trail crossed into the Anaconda–Pintler Wilderness, traversed the south face of Mount Tiny, and then topped out on Goat Flat, a broad expanse of alpine tundra. The Anaconda Cutoff ended on top of the plateau, where our trail met the official CDT coming in from Upper Seymour Lake. After crossing the delicate tundra, we dropped through larch forest. Farther on we paused at an unsigned intersection that matched nothing on our map. After 20 minutes of walking we decided we'd chosen the wrong fork. Backtracking, we followed the other trail to quiet Flower Lake and set up camp for the night.

The concept of a "trail" is an interesting one to consider in the context of long-distance hiking. Several long-distance hikers we met—particularly those who had walked the Appalachian Trail—thought that the Continental Divide Trail should be, well . . . a little more "trail-like." By that they meant that intersections should be signed and that the tread should always be clearly distinguishable.

The trouble isn't that long-distance hikers lack the skills to read the landscape and use a map and compass. What long-distance hikers generally lack is *time*. A couple of missed trails here or half-day mistakes there can extend the journey dangerously close to winter. Every day, every minute, every mile, every step is precious. Traveling only across Montana, Kate and I did not feel the time crunch nearly as acutely as our compatriots who were walking the entire 3,100 miles of the CDT.

We were initially surprised to learn of many long-distance hikers' near-total devotion to Jim Wolf's CDT hiking guides. Jim Wolf runs the Continental Divide Trail Society, an organization dedicated to the planning, development, and maintenance of the CDT as a silent trail. Because of his advocacy for the trail and his excellent guidebooks, many hikers think of Wolf as the "father" of the CDT. Wolf's guidebooks are exhaustive, giving trail descriptions down to the tenth of a mile. Details might include the shape of a gnarled knot on a trailside tree or the number of stepping-stones across a small creek. His preciseness led Kate to frequently say of Wolf, "I just love his nerdlike enthusiasm." For us, Wolf's book had actually been a late throw-in. We could have managed all of our hiking in the northern half of Montana with large grained maps and maybe a compass reading or two. But later, in the remote southwest corner of the state, Wolf's guide would prove invaluable, particularly in pointing out water sources.

For much of three days we roller-coastered through the heart of the

Pintlers: up to Rainbow Saddle, Cutaway Pass, and Warner Lake; down into Queener Basin and LaMarche and Fishtrap Creeks. The high points revealed saw-toothed peaks, jagged ridgelines, talus* slopes, and immense alpine plateaus stretching away in all directions. In the valleys, we crossed through forests of whitebark pine, spruce, and fir.

Carrying over a week's worth of food, I finished each day tired and sore, as tired and sore as I had been the entire trip. Kate, in the meantime, motored strongly, having no residual blister problem and, thankfully, no dizziness. Since her cancer treatments, low red blood cell counts have been a constant problem for Kate. The climbs and descents through the Pintlers mostly occur over 8,000 feet, plus we crossed the 9,000-foot level for the first time of the hike. We felt blessed that Kate registered no light-headedness.

On our third day in the Pintlers we rested and ate lunch at Rainbow Lake. The massive form of West Goat Peak towered over the lake like a pyramid climbing out of the desert. A quick climb to Rainbow Pass revealed more beauty on the west side of the Divide. Aquamarine Martin and Johnson Lakes sat serenely in front of East Pintler Peak. Emerald forests bathed the valleys; chunky clouds, white and unthreatening, played against the solid wall of the Divide. Warm sunshine and a slight west wind pulled Kate and me into the scene. For 20 minutes, little more than three or four words passed between us.

At Johnson Lake we camped near two friendly women from Missoula. Patricia, the older of the two, had silver hair and spoke fondly of her attempt to hike the full CDT years earlier. Sarah was a quiet, striking woman originally from Atlanta. For a time Sarah lay quietly in the grass while Patricia described her approach to hiking the Continental Divide, plus what she liked and disliked about various pieces of backpacking equipment.

At dusk I broke away to fish, taking a number of wild cutthroats that were rising to crane flies. Kate, Sarah, and Patricia were by then engaged in a lively discussion. I yelled excitedly when I landed my first fish, a golden treasure to behold. "Yee-haw, I caught one! Does anyone want to see it?"

*Rock debris.

Patricia answered from the other side of the trees, "Is it exceptionally big?"

"Well, no, not really."

"Is it exceedingly small?"

"No!"

"Well, we don't need to see it then. We've all seen fish, thank you." My ego shattered, I did not announce my subsequent catches.

Morning yoga helped to revive my sore muscles. After breakfast, Sarah and Patricia decided to accompany us to Oreamnos Lake. The four of us passed through larch forest and sunlit openings covered with wild-flowers. Patricia pointed out elephant-head and parrot's beak. Near Pintler Pass, entire meadows glowed lupine purple. Though it was mid-August, there at 9,000 feet some of the lupine had only just flowered.

We parted from these excellent companions at Oreamnos Lake. Kate and I walked to the opposite end of the lake, then up the inlet creek. Thousands of red monkey flowers overwhelmed the small waterway. Soon the path, a faint line in the grass, climbed straight up a rugged shoulder of West Pintler Peak. The track disappeared as we dropped pre-cipitously into Sawed Cabin Lake, then reappeared as the big peaks of the Anaconda–Pintler began to fall behind us. The more rounded terrain before us led to a softer tread—a welcome relief after the hard rock and scrabble offered to that point in the Pintlers.

Unable to find a suitable camp along the Divide trail, Kate and I took a mile side trip down to Mystic Lake. Just before making the turn, we spot-ted a gold-brown fisher perched in a tree. The singular beast, the size of a well-fed housecat, stared at us without fear, its eyes large and ears inqui-sitive.

The lake stood deserted. We cooked dinner on the veranda of the Forest Service patrol cabin as hail pounded the roof. In the morning fog blanketed the lake's surface. An early sun cut though the forest, sending daggers of light into the mist. Overhead, blue sky welcomed the day as the fog grudgingly dissipated. Smoky wisps hovered over the lake, swirling with the breeze like ghosts in a B movie. Suddenly, out of the depths of the centuries, an eerie howl sounded, at first short and then in a long, deep, reverberating voice.

Kate's eyes caught mine. Without conviction, she whispered, "Loon?"

As the howl's pitch rose, we answered her question in tandem, "Wolf."

The howl continued from directly across the lake, a lone voice calling out to the mountains. The cold morning air froze with the majesty of the cry. We sat silent and awestruck, tingling.*

◩

We made a couple of sad discoveries during that summer of recovery. The first, as I've already described, was that Kate could no longer eat a number of foods without becoming gravely ill. Suddenly eating at restaurants and at friends' houses became difficult. Kate constantly struggled to balance culinary gratification against potential abdominal pain. While she has learned much about her digestive system, gastrointestinal pain from acidic foods or hidden milk products continues to plague her to this day.

The second discovery—a diagnosis of lymphedema—was something we'd been struggling with since Kate's original radical hysterectomy. Periodically throughout our summer of recovery, Kate's legs grew abnormally heavy. Kate was thin-legged to start with, so even when they were swollen, her legs generally received little comment from our doctors. "They look pretty good to me," the doctors would say to her complaints. But to Kate, an athlete used to running and biking for hours on end, the sudden heaviness of her calves and thighs caused misery. Many times she complained that swelling made her ankles and knees stiff, and that swollen thighs left her feeling that she couldn't lift her legs high enough to run. Once when I talked about entering a marathon again, Kate cried.

---

*Gray wolves were extirpated from the Northern Rockies by the 1930s. Unlike in Yellowstone National Park and the central Idaho wilderness complex, no wolf reintroductions have occurred in the Pintlers. Transient populations appear to exist, however. David Dorian, the Sula postmaster, described to us seeing a wolf on the edge of the Pintler Range. Norm Bishop, a retired wolf specialist from Yellowstone Park, suggests that the wolf we heard most likely dispersed from one of the introduced central Idaho packs. As the crow flies, it is only 40 miles from Mystic Lake to the edge of the "Selway Pack's" home range. Forty miles, according to Norm, is little distance for a wolf to travel, especially given few intervening roads. Additionally, since the original Selway reintroduction of 35 animals has grown to roughly 150, it's reasonable to believe that a dispersing pressure exists.

Norm also noted two reasons that the central Idaho packs are likely to disperse greater distances than the Yellowstone packs. First, to acclimate wolves to their surroundings before release,

As that summer of recovery turned into fall and then fall slid into the years ahead, we worked hard to create positives out of Kate's new limitations. Though a healthy eater before the cancer, Kate eats an almost exclusively vegan diet now and, to some extent, I do the same. We also now regularly juice fresh vegetables to drink. We've changed to buying organic foods whenever possible. Science doesn't always know the effect of *de minimis* quantities of pesticides on the human body. Regardless, Kate and I know that her immune system remains depressed and needs no unnecessary challenges. We also know that pesticides are tough on the environment. And so, in a strange way, cancer has improved us.

Cancer has led to other positives in our lives. Kate's lymphedema, for example, led us to a new form of exercise: swimming. The relative weightlessness, prone positioning, and water pressure of swimming minimize the gravity-pulling, lymph-settling forces of running. Additionally, swimming is a lifelong exercise that induces fewer joint and muscle injuries than running. Sure, Kate still runs—shorter distances these days—but cancer brought swimming into our lives.

◤

By the time Kate and I hiked away from Mystic Lake, the fog and the wolf had disappeared. It was mid-August, yet the midmorning air retained a cold edge. A few days earlier, we had seen a bull elk heavy with solid antlers. I zipped my turtleneck and wondered out loud if the chill wasn't the first hint of fall.

We climbed back to the CDT and followed it directly along the spine of the continent. Through breaks in the forest we could see the Big Hole

---

biologists held the Yellowstone packs in pens for ten weeks. The central Idaho packs were simply driven to the end of a road and released. Second, in Yellowstone, biologists made an effort to create packs during the acclimatization time (e.g., pairing adults). This effort was not made in central Idaho.

It's interesting to note that southwest Montana's Continental Divide wildlands, though not federally designated wilderness, provide a nearly continuous wildlife corridor between central Idaho and Yellowstone National Park. Conceivably, wolves (plus grizzly bears and other animals) might someday again move along that corridor. To keep that possibility open, the lands must be protected.

Valley close at hand, and behind that the Pioneer Mountains. Further east stood the Tobacco Roots and south from there the Snowcrest and Gravelly Ranges. Nearer—to the west and abutting the Divide—we could make out massive Squaw Mountain and Homer Youngs Peak in the Bitterroot Range. South from them stood Baldy Mountain, Cottonwood and Italian and the Red Conglomerate Peaks, and then finally the Centennials leading into Yellowstone National Park. The entirety of southwest Montana stood in front of us, rimmed by the Continental Divide like a giant C-clamp meant for squeezing water into the Missouri River's upper drainages.

Kate and I gawked a bit at the scene before us, realizing that walking around Montana's southwest "corner" meant a chance to explore another 350 miles of inspiring country. We felt flush with anticipation, yet also saddened. Both of us realized that not one step along the entire remainder of our path would be through protected wilderness. Once we walked out of the Anaconda–Pintler Wilderness later that day, we were back in the Old West of Montana, a world of extractive industries and motorized recreation and don't-tell-me-what-to-do mentalities.

By mid-afternoon we reached an intersection. A bold map and sign declared the CDT closed due to wildfire. We had been curious about recent helicopter activity, but had seen no smoke. Kate and I had planned to camp at Surprise Lake that night, which according to the posted map was in the center of the fire zone. We spent an embarrassingly long time discussing whether we should proceed anyway. How bad could the fire be? In the end the threatened $5,000 fine and six months in jail carried the day. We couldn't finish the hike if we were sitting in the clink.

So we turned onto the trail to Mussigbrod Lake to circumvent the fire zone. The change in route would take us off the Divide, add miles to our hike, and require a fair amount of cross-country travel. Kate groused a little, fairly certain that with commando tactics she could have eluded any serious time in the pen. I asked her what our motto was when things went bad. I expected to hear something reflective, something like, "We do the best with wherever we are, with whatever life hands us." That philosophy, though trite, had brought us through many days of cancer treatment. In the hospital, Kate ill, we couldn't run or go outside. Still we could read out loud to each other, something we truly enjoy. And so we would read.

But instead Kate shouted into the forest, "Our motto is, *let it burn!*" I laughed and Kate smiled, though somewhat weakly. Kate has often given me a hard time for my endlessly optimistic outlook on life. Hence, it came as no surprise when she followed with, "Just let me say, 'This *sucks*,' for an hour, okay? Then I'll be fine."

After that, the walk away from the Divide passed pleasantly, easily. A cow moose moved off the trail in front of us, just a few steps into dense lodgepole. She stood silently as we passed, her head pivoting 180 degrees to follow our progress. We stopped at the campground on Mussigbrod Lake, where other campers confirmed that helicopters had been flying the ridge for days, apparently fighting a fire in the Dense Creek drainage across the Divide.

For much of the next two days we walked along nonexistent or hidden trail. From Mussigbrod Lake we struck out overland to Bender Creek, following our compass as we rounded the fire zone. In the end we emerged from the forest at the bend of a quiet road, exactly as shown on our map.

We hiked on in a light drizzle and soon turned back to the Divide on a road along Johnson Creek. After climbing for a couple of hours, we cut a long switchback, passing through a recent clear-cut. There, 30 yards before Schultz Saddle, we discovered a CDT reassurance symbol! As one we yelled theatrically, "We're *back on*, baby!" It's funny what a good friend the trail had become, almost as if it had a spirit of its own—something to cherish and look forward to, a companion in its own right.

After tossing away two elk forelegs, Kate and I set up for the night in an abandoned hunters' camp. We sipped mint tea while we cooked, content that we had successfully navigated our way around the fire, that we felt warm in the late sun, and that a night of reading aloud awaited. As importantly, we felt blessed that our feet had finally recovered from the running shoe debacle, and that the following night we would soak in a hot springs.

Rigorous physical effort yields satisfaction from the smallest things. Simplicity breeds contentment.

◢

A friend once asked if the process of healing from cancer meant being able to both accept and ignore the cancer. The question showed great perception. While we have accepted the reality of cancer and the limitations it has brought to our lives, throughout our cancer experience Kate has found ways to ignore the horror and get on with her life.

Even in the hospital, the ability to focus ahead—on her treatments and on getting well—turned Kate's mind away from cancer. "I had a treatment plan set out for me by my doctors," Kate explained. "That helped me just look at one step at a time. I'd say to myself, 'Just get through the next treatment. I know everything isn't great right now, but I'm going along with the plan and it is going to work.'"

Kate created positive stress to push her beyond expectations. While in the hospital, she fought to take a shower when no one thought her strong enough, or pushed to walk farther than the doctors suggested she might. "It felt so good," Kate later related, "to accomplish a goal." Kate worked on learning Spanish and oversaw our investments right from the hospital bed, all in an effort to regain her sense of self.

At home, during the days of agonizing waits between doctors' appointments, Kate further focused on recovering her autonomy. "I think it helps incredibly to keep doing some regular activities," Kate told me. "If I could feel like I accomplished something in a day like paying bills, cooking dinner, or going on my longest walk yet, then I could feel human and hopeful. If I had let everything be done for me, I would have felt like I was getting the message to give up. I think you had to take care of a lot more responsibilities because I didn't have energy. But it was important that I was needed to do some things as well."

During our summer of recovery, I often sounded the voice of caution. We seemed to be pushing, pushing, pushing, as if these were our last chances ever to be in wild country together. I asked Kate if kayaking alone through remote Pacific islands or canoeing alone down rivers unknown to us really made sense. Those journeys would have been challenging enough for us, I argued, even with her at full strength.

Nothing I said, however, deterred Kate's desire to climb back into her life. "It might be hard, but we can make it," was about the most I ever extracted from her.

I saw this dogged mindset so often, I started calling it Kate's "no-excuses" attitude. Instead of making excuses for what she couldn't do, she pushed hard to accomplish those things she could.

◪

Even after circumventing the fire, our trials with hidden trails were not over. From Schultz Saddle, Old Trail #110 had been renamed CDT #9, but little else had been done in years. The trail frequently disappeared into new clear-cuts. Picking up the tread on the far side of ten acres of mowed trees proved exceedingly difficult. We probably added two hours to our hike the next day searching for, and eventually always finding, the trail. Unfortunately, even what trail existed suffered from great neglect. Deadfall continuously interrupted the track.

Kate and I opted to follow a side trail rather than stay on the Divide since we wanted to see the Hogan Creek Forest Service cabin along Trail Creek.

The area is rife with history. Lost Trail Pass—a few miles ahead and our day's destination—was named when Lewis and Clark's Indian guide, Old Toby, became lost nearby. On the return east from the Pacific, after separating from Lewis to follow a southerly route, Clark passed through the valley Kate and I now walked. He and his men had crossed the Divide at what was later named Gibbons Pass, in honor of Lieutenant Colonel John Gibbon. In 1877, Lieutenant Gibbon and his battalion chased Chief Joseph and his Nez Percé band across that same pass. Shortly thereafter, a few miles east from there near Wisdom, the Nez Percé survived a surprise attack by the U.S. Army. The Army was attempting to force the band of roughly 800 Indians onto a reservation in the western Idaho Territory. Rather than submit to the federal government's demands, the Nez Percé chose to flee their ancestral homelands in the Columbia Basin. The chase ran for four months from eastern Oregon to the Bear Paw Mountains just south of present-day Havre, Montana.

Rather than follow Trail Creek as Captain Clark, Colonel Gibbon, and

Chief Joseph had, Kate and I climbed out of the valley and walked roads from Hogan Cabin to Lost Trail Pass. Arriving at the pass, we felt euphoric. Only once more before the end of our hike across Montana—at Monida—did we plan a break from the trail. The hike's end, though still distant, now seemed truly reachable.

First things first, though: We had to cover the six or eight miles from Lost Trail Pass to Lost Trail Hot Springs, where we planned to take a day and a half off. Kate and I had two ride offers before we even stuck out our thumbs. Happily, the man we hooked up with turned out to be Gordon Reese of the Continental Divide Trail Alliance (CDTA).

It turns out that CDTA volunteers had just finished a weekend work party around Gibbons Pass. We had missed that trail section because of our desire to see Hogan Cabin. Indeed, the trail crew had stayed at Hogan Cabin the night before we arrived there. Gordon asked if we had run into Jim Wolf, *the* Jim Wolf of Continental Divide Trail Society (CDTS) and guidebook fame. According to Gordon, Wolf was mapping trail changes in the area and had been at the pass just 30 minutes before us.

Although we were sad that we missed Wolf, Kate and I felt lucky to have met Gordon. Gordon explained that the CDTA is a nonprofit group dedicated to protecting, promoting, constructing, and managing a primitive trail along the Continental Divide. If Jim Wolf of the CDTS is the father of the Continental Divide Trail, then the CDTA must certainly be its caring family (and most prominent advocates). While Wolf maps the trail, members of the CDTA, behind their dynamic and dedicated leaders Bruce and Paula Ward, work on the ground to improve it.*

By the time he dropped us off at Lost Trail Hot Springs, Gordon had given us CDTA membership information and a leftover care package from the trail crew party. Kate and I spent a full rest day at Lost Trail Hot Springs doing laundry, soaking in the pools, and collecting our mail and food at nearby Sula. David Dorian, the postmaster at Sula, was expecting us. David's entire building wasn't much bigger than a postage stamp. Thus our two food boxes took up a substantial percentage of his available space.

*In 1997 the CDTA was designated the lead non-governmental organization for interacting with federal agencies on matters of the CDT. Also noteworthy, the CDTA has recently started publishing its own trail guides to the CDT.

After organizing the food behind the post office, Kate and I hitched a ride back to Lost Trail Hot Springs. Once there, we settled into the soothing pools as shadows moved across the valley. While we luxuriated, Kate informed me smartly that Lewis and Clark had actually *missed* Lost Trail Hot Springs.

"Really?" I marveled.

Fanning the smoky waters in front of her, my chief guide continued, "We're obviously on the better trip."

◪

Kate and I sat in front of the tent, this time in northwestern British Columbia. We were in the midst of our summer of recovery, on a nine-day canoe trip down a wild river. I had portaged the canoe and gear five kilometers to the put-in because Kate was not strong enough to carry much.

Just what we thought we were doing, I'm not sure. We were only four months out from Kate's bowel resection surgery and still uncertain about the stability of her health. In nine days we would see people only twice. If Kate ran into medical problems, we would just have to work them out on our own, deep in the backcountry. In a lot of ways that canoe trip symbolized our burning desire to make a break from the medical world. We desperately needed the confidence to take care of ourselves again.

Our tent sat near the river, on the open cobble of a wide inside corner. I was reading Barry Lopez's *Of Wolves and Men*:

> Wolves and prey may remain absolutely still while staring at each other. . . . An intense stare is frequently used by wolves to communicate with each other, and wolves also tend to engage strangers—wolf and human—in stares. I think what transpires in those moments of staring is an exchange of information between predator and prey that either triggers a chase or diffuses the hunt right there. I call this exchange the conversation of death. . . .

I had, incredibly, just read this passage when I looked up and saw a jet-black wolf coming up the river, right over Kate's shoulder. I whispered to

Kate and we both turned to watch the wolf amble toward us—closer, then closer still. At 25 paces the wolf stopped, its fiery eyes intent on us.

For a moment there was nothing, and then Kate said, "Good wolf, go away wolf."

The stare continued. Then the wolf broke toward us in two aggressive bounds. We stayed solid and on the third bound the wolf cut off into the willows, and disappeared.

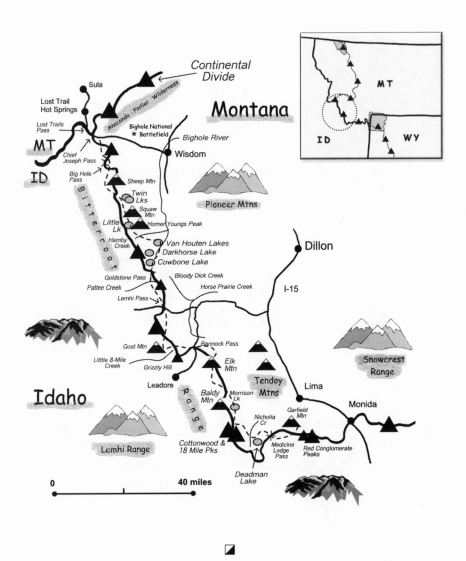

Our hiking route **(Chapters 10 and 11)** from Chief Joseph Pass on the edge of the Pintlers south and east to Garfield Mountain west of I-15. Our route is shown as a dashed line. The inset shows the approximate area included in the larger map.

TEN

Facing Into the Current

. . . I had accomplished one of those great objects
on which my mind has been unalterably fixed for many years,
judge then of the pleasure I felt in allying my thirst
with this pure and ice cold water.

CAPTAIN MERIWETHER LEWIS
upon first crossing the Continental Divide at Lemhi Pass
as quoted in *Undaunted Courage* by Stephen Ambrose

KATE AND I stuffed our packs full of 11 days worth of food and then joined Ray, the salty owner of the Lost Trail Hot Springs, for breakfast at the lodge. Ray cussed the bicycle tourists who camped with him the previous night—30 folks who negotiated a cheap group rate, then filled his dumpsters with garbage from a huge barbeque party and never ate a single meal at his restaurant.

"People don't know how expensive garbage is, hauling it down the valley and all," Ray muttered.

A moment later Ray nodded to a couple of young fellows cleaning the pools, noting that many of the kids working for him came from Job Corps. Some of the kids had stolen from him and one had wrecked his car, Ray told us.

"But the program's important, the kids have got to get on their feet somehow." Ray was an ornery curmudgeon with a heart about a mile wide.

Ray kindly offered Kate and me a ride back up to the CDT where we'd left off at Lost Trail Pass. We had barely bid him farewell and started for Chief Joseph Pass when Kate's bowels began to cramp. We could only guess she had accidentally ingested a milk product. Kate soon moaned in distress. She quickly took a pain pill—the first pain pill she'd taken in recent memory.

"It reminds me that I used to feel this way every day," Kate said somberly.

The pain pill eased Kate's discomfort and we started again. Seven miles down the trail we found water. We decided to make a short day of it and eat up some food weight. Since we had seen only two people all day, Kate and I set up camp on the ridge top, just alongside the gravel road we had been walking on. Slashes of plum-colored clouds loomed over the mountains to the west. Sheets of shimmering rain and shafts of sunlight slanted down from the heavens. Later an orange sunset burned on the horizon, coloring the smoke of distant fires in Idaho.

A beautiful sunset, still air, and silence. It is as difficult to describe the peace and contentedness of a long-distance hike as it is to ignore it. Just then, camped beside a lonely road, in a place we might never otherwise consider, we felt happy and at peace. We felt the importance of what life was at that moment providing us: a drink of cold water, a soft place to sleep, a full stomach, tingling muscles, and cool, clean air. Gone were the daily onslaughts of marketing messages telling us we needed more, more, more. How different it was to simply say, "I am happy. I have enough."

It's interesting to consider what brings on such a state of contentment. The endless time to think? The physical effort of the hike? The reconnection of mind and body? The simplicity of carrying only what you can use? The mountains and trees and sagebrush and moose? It was all of those things and more. The *more* for us was a willingness to live here and now and accept what God had given us. The *more* was a willingness to focus on the multitude of blessings we had, rather than on how life had shorted us.

◪

Reality truly is what we see and, maybe more importantly, what we allow ourselves to see.

Walking along through the forest one day, Kate and I learned that lesson from a spruce grouse. For the most part, spruce grouse are considered dumber than stones, a thought reflected in their nickname, "fool hens." As you approach them, these birds typically stand in the trail or sit on a branch, so calm and unfettered that a hurled rock could easily kill them. Fool hens seem genetically programmed to serve as emergency meals for lost hikers.

So how then do fool hens survive? Camouflage provides the only possible answer.

Ahead of me, alongside the trail, stood a fool hen like so many we had already seen. The fool hen's mottled plumage blended in so well with the thin undergrowth that I would have never seen the bird had she not clucked.

I waved at Kate to walk up slowly. For fully a minute we watched the still bird, just three feet in front of us. Then, as Kate and I started to leave, the ground around the hen suddenly *moved*—two chicks rattled awkwardly away.

We had only allowed ourselves to see the undergrowth. The chicks had been four inches from their mother the entire time we had been staring at her.

◪

From Yellowstone Park north to Chief Joseph Pass, the Continental Divide forms the border between Montana and Idaho. At Chief Joseph Pass, however, the state boundary and the Divide part company; the state boundary turns southwest while the Divide heads northeast.

As a Montana kid I always heard that the Montana border had been intended to follow the Divide north from Chief Joseph Pass. As the story went, some early surveyors had mistaken the Bitterroot Range for the Divide, a blunder that led to residents of present-day Missoula and Kalispell filling out Montana rather than Idaho tax forms.

This story is not true, says Bill Cunningham in his book *Montana's Continental Divide*. He writes that Sidney Edgerton, an Eastern politician who was soon to be the Montana territory's first governor, politicked his way to the land grab. Early on, the Idaho Territory included today's Montana, Idaho, and Wyoming. By the 1860s many realized that Lewiston, the Idaho Territory capital, was too far away to govern the miners and merchants pouring into southwest Montana. The Idaho contingency argued for territory separation along the Continental Divide. Edgerton, an acquaintance of President Lincoln and a friend to the chairman of the House Committee on Territories, set his sights on more land for the new Montana territory, and he got it.

Kate and I were walking just then on the *un*disputed section of the border that Edgerton had haggled over, the section that crawled right along the crest of the Divide. South of Chief Joseph Pass, we came upon rock cairns with metal pipes sticking up from their centers. These state line markers, which we would follow for much of the next 300 miles, had caps forged with an M | I imprint. The raised letters, interestingly, did not always indicate the states on their proper sides.

We followed the Divide through wild country. A bull elk, a bull moose, and immense Douglas firs added to the sense of remoteness. We spent a night at Big Hole Pass, then another on the South Fork of Sheep Creek, where forest fire smoke hung heavily in the treetops. The smoke transformed stately Sheep Mountain into a hazy phantom hovering over our tent.

I purified water not far up the trail from our camp. On the opposite side of the spring from where I sat, a tiny spider walked its gossamer web up and down, checking and rechecking numerous trapped mayflies. I could smell smoke. I grew reflective, as I did every night while I pumped our water supply. What, I wondered, would Kate and I do if a fire rushed through this forested valley? At last report, the main fire complex was many miles distant, yet if strong winds suddenly pushed it our way would we be able to move fast enough to stay ahead of the flames? We were deep in the wilderness with no ready escape route. We could only hope for friendly winds and trust in our abilities to sense danger in time to act.

I pushed Kate for a 6:30 A.M. start the next day to better tackle some tough bushwhacking we expected just ahead. Kate moaned a bit at my early morning revelry. Referring to Ray Jardine, the infamous lightweight hiking aficionado who claims to often rise before sunrise, I told her, "Hey you should feel lucky—the Gear Nazi would have you up at 4:30."

Kate groaned and then pulled the sleeping bag over her head. From underneath came a muffled, "That guy must be totally obnoxious to hike with."

Sometimes it's nice when the guidebooks are out of date. The bushwhacking we expected that day proved nonexistent. Instead, after leaving the South Fork of Sheep Creek, we found a brilliant new trail switchbacking up to the head of Fourth of July Creek. Crossing the Divide, we left most of the previous day's smoke behind. Twin Lakes, flanked by the Big Hole Valley, sparkled like two sapphires below us to the east. Ahead, more southerly, the imposing hulk of Squaw Mountain waited. Kate and I walked on, joyous and alone through outstanding country.

We spent a cold night at Slag-a-Melt Lakes and then climbed a scant trail out of the basin. For 10 or 15 miles there in the Bitterroots the CDT runs parallel to the Divide proper, meaning it runs perpendicular to the drainages. We climbed ridges, passed delicate tarns, and then dropped into deep valleys. Once we swung wide around a glacial moraine before crossing a pretty creek. The trail then passed through open meadows with scattered groups of pines, large granite outcroppings, and thousands of purple gentians. Ahead, a sheer rock face rose straight up out of the south side of Little Lake. The other side of the lake, where we would set our tent, held a flat meadow lush with grass and wildflowers. Homer Youngs Peak guarded the lake's eastern flank while the Divide formed a towering backdrop to the west.

Trout dimpled Little Lake's surface as the sun dropped behind the Divide. The cutthroats greedily accepted my flies, but soon a cold air mass dropping into the basin drove us to the tent. At 2 A.M. I climbed back out of the tent to a sky filled with stars, interrupted only on the western horizon by the dark silhouette of the Divide. By 6:30 A.M., the temperature in the tent had dropped to 37 degrees. In the meadow, the gentians had all folded tight against the late summer's first frost.

Hot tea and morning yoga warmed Kate and me as we waited for the sun to clear Homer Youngs Peak. High above Little Lake, four mountain goats walked along a ridge in the sunshine. Their white coats phosphoresced against the charcoal talus backdrop. Later, after we crawled up to the ridge, I crossed a rocky outcrop in search of the goats but could not find them.

By day's end we had passed Rock Island Lakes, climbed up the steep ridge of the Miner Basin, and dropped through second growth forest to set up camp near Hamby Creek. Along the way Kate had a close encounter with a cow elk that did not want to yield the trail. More cows—the bovine variety—filled the meadows along Hamby Creek. A healthy riparian zone suggested that the cows had not been there long.

With the tent up, Kate and I walked in search of a beaver pond, then returned to camp to read aloud and build one of our infrequent fires in an existing fire pit. Warming her hands at the fire, Kate looked at me mischievously.

"I know you're doing more work than me on this trip—putting up the tent, pumping the water, doing the dishes—but it's okay," she assured me. "The balance is so incredibly out of whack at home the other way, I'll just let you have this chance to catch up."

Egging her on, I replied, "Well, we could skip the nightly leg massages."

"But you do those at home anyway!"

"I'm just happy to be with you," I said with a shrug.

Kate gave me a smile and turned away to grab something. I stared into the fire. My heart rose to my throat and I felt a tear roll down my cheek.

◪

As the end of our summer of recovery approached, Kate began to express a desire to return to work. Additionally, her long-term disability agreement with Hewlett-Packard—though modifiable—stated that she would be back in mid-September. I argued for Kate to extend her leave, thinking that the longer she could delay the stress of work the better off she would be. But Kate demurred. Throughout the summer of travel and outdoor living, she had grown stronger day by day. Her weight had increased and her hair, though still curly, was lengthening. We had not been at work in over ten months. Kate declared that it was time to get back to our normal lives.

Kate decided to work only half-time when she returned to HP in September of 1995. I returned to work full-time. Both of us were kindly welcomed back by our managers and work compatriots.

Kate's half-time status lasted a couple of months, a time during which she struggled to bike the three miles between our house and the HP campus. The biking reflected Kate's dogged stubbornness about controlling her return to health. "If I'm well enough to work," she argued, "I'm well enough to bike to work." She frequently arrived home at night tired and drained.

Though not at full strength, Kate soon became immersed in an important work project. By Christmas she decided to return to work full-time. While tiring, returning to work full-time held a certain allure: certainly that would prove that Kate's life had returned to normal. Before long she was traveling one week every month. But every time the work routine began to set in, we would have to put everything on hold to return to Seattle for Kate's regular checkup. Departing Corvallis, we would draw in a collective breath, realizing that what we learned in Seattle could reverse the course of our lives in a single moment.

As the months of full-time work wore on, Kate had an enlightening revelation: She no longer wanted her "normal" life to be defined by her work life. I shared that revelation. We had joined a lunchtime reading group at work, and often the group's book selections focused on the disconnect between a person's work life and his or her life's work. In *The Heart Aroused,* poet David Whyte describes the disconnect like this:

> . . . you must look hard at the road you are taking now as much as the hoped-for destination. You must admit what you see on that road and grieve long for what you do not. Then you have a possibility of waking.

Our passion for the world outside work was nothing new, but Kate's revelation brought a new approach to that passion. As quickly as she could arrange it, Kate cut down permanently to a four-day, 32-hour workweek. Not long after, I did the same. Having Fridays free provided a chance for Kate to rest and rebound from work stress, a chance for us to explore Oregon, a chance to dream. Recovering some of our time meant reclaiming some of ourselves. We felt revitalized. Again, David Whyte:

> *The river down which we raft*
> *is made up of the same substance*
> *as the great sea of our destination.*

◪

At Berry Creek, the CDT turned downstream and dropped away from the Divide. We followed the road along the creek and spooked a young moose out of some willows. Farther on we emerged from the forest and started out into flat sagebrush country. Soon we heard the putt-putt of a fat-tired, one-person motor scooter slowly approaching from behind.

The OHV rider was remarkable for two reasons. First, because he drove slowly; and second, because his dog, a golden retriever, sat comfortably perched on the OHV's rear rack. A rifle scabbard was mounted to the OHV's frame, but on this day a fishing rod protruded from it. The OHVer was an older fellow, wearing a camouflage hat, jean shirt, and working-man's boots. The man killed the motor, swung his leg over his machine, and introduced himself as Duane Ehrenberg from Dillon.

It was hard not to notice that Duane wore a sidearm. For his part, Duane couldn't believe we hiked without a gun, with bears and cougars and the like about. We told him that in known grizzly country, like Glacier National Park, we carried pepper spray.

"Pepper spray? Huh!" Duane huffed incredulously. "Don't you know they paint-mark problem grizzlies and then drop them in a place like this?" We told him we didn't know that.*

"Me, I wouldn't go anywhere in these woods without a gun. That's why I got this little baby." Here Duane mistakenly gestured to his folding pliers tool rather than the Colt .45 that also hung from his belt. I thought

---

*Arnold Dood at Montana Fish, Wildlife, and Parks confirmed my belief that no such program exists.

Duane might launch into a tirade then, but instead he softened. "I don't want to shoot 'em," he laughed, "jus' scare 'em enough so that I can get up a tree! Place like Glacier, griz attacks a person up there and then it's the bear that ends up getting killed. That don't seem right. I like griz—my dog's named Griz."

Duane expressed further astonishment when Kate told him we were hiking Montana's Continental Divide. "You say your rig's in Monida. And you're walkin' from here to there. Jeesh!" Duane shook his head is disbelief. "You must write for *National Geographic* or *Reader's Digest* or something like that." Though we claimed otherwise, Duane insisted we give him our names so he could look for us in future editions.

Duane and Griz putted slowly away, but an hour later we came across them again, on the road. Duane leaned out the window of his pickup to ask a question, "Don't ya sometimes jus' git a hankerin' for a good steak?"

After a pregnant pause, Duane furrowed his eyebrows and then slowly drawled, "Or are you both veg-ee-tarians?"

We all laughed and then Duane said, "Do you know what you two need?"

No dummy, I answered simultaneously with him, "A beer!"

Duane and Griz drove away a few moments later, leaving Kate and me to walk on, cold beers in hand, puzzling over people. I have an intense dislike of OHVs in wildlands, admitted. But Duane reminded us that people who approach life from different angles can still be just plain good folk.

A melodic blend of lowing cows and howling coyotes welcomed dawn the following morning at Van Houten Lake. Two ducks came in over the treetops, wings whistling like miniature jet fighters. A beaver left a long V in the placid lake. Kate and I rose cold again, then took immense joy in a pot of billy tea* before starting upstream along the diminishing Big Hole River.

By the time we reached Skinner Meadows, the sun had taken hold of the day. Far out in the grass two sandhill cranes, looking ever so much like pterodactyls of old, rattled through a croaky, staccato call.

---

*Kiwis and Aussies historically made tea in a pot or a can called a "billy" when camping in the bush. "Billy tea" is a term Kate and I picked up during a year we spent Down Under. We've been using it ever since.

We turned up the road to Darkhorse Mine and climbed back toward the Divide. After a steep ascent along a cascading creek, we topped out on a bench, crossed a rutted jeep road, and found beautiful Darkhorse Lake nestled directly under the peaks of the Divide.

Sadly, my demeanor toward OHV riders, which had softened a bit because of our talks with Duane, suddenly turned rock hard. Darkhorse Lake had been decimated. It could have served as the poster child for everything wrong with allowing motorized vehicles into pristine lands. A quagmire of mud and ruts, tire tracks, and torn earth surrounded the lake. The ratty foreshore held little vegetation other than trees. Garbage littered the area: broken bottles, beer cans, candy wrappers, cigarette butts, Styrofoam plates, clay pigeons, old tables, and metal grates.

The desecration made our blood run cold. We recalled less than a week earlier peering into a serene valley in the Bitterroots, only to have the peace shattered by racing OHV motors. We soon spotted a mucky road and on it two OHVs shooting rooster tails of mud at every corner. We remembered in other places locked gates that OHV riders had simply circumvented through the woods, and all through Montana ugly trails eroded and widened by the big-treaded tires. And we recalled once hearing an off-road enthusiast claim that OHVs weren't a "problem," but rather just part of the "natural progression" of things. From foot, to horse, to OHV—clearly a simple extension of Darwinian evolution.

Looking at the devastation in front of us, it was hard for Kate and me not to see irony in our nightly concern over crushing delicate grasses and wildflowers with the tent.

Saddened, we hiked the short distance to Cowbone Lake, so named for a herd of cattle that died there after collapsing through thin ice. The rutted road plowed on in that direction, so we expected more of the same and were disappointed not to be disappointed. As we arrived, two motorcyclists climbed onto their machines. The men said they had a camp back at Darkhorse Lake. They talked about fishing and introduced us to their kids, who climbed onto the machines behind them.

"It's a dads' weekend," one of the men said. "We left the women at home."

Alone, then, Kate and I picked up hordes of broken glass and pitched them in the only place available to us, an immense fire pit. When later a tent pole connector went askew, I swore angrily, working on it for several fruitless minutes. Bemused, Kate calmly took the pole from me and, within moments, magically repaired it.

Handing the pole back, she remarked dryly, "Good thing you didn't leave 'the women' at home."

◪

To regain the Divide the following morning, we had to sidehill through loose, slippery shingle, then climb vertically on poor trail. Though she spotted a mountain goat along the way, Kate disliked this kind of hiking and her mood soured considerably.

Much of Kate's discomfort came from the difficulty of lifting her legs. Sometimes she complained that her muscle tone had never completely returned after the five surgeries. Also, the tight leggings she wore to battle lymphedema restricted her knees from bending, creating a struggle akin to hiking in neoprene waders. When Kate's legs swelled, as they had during many of the hot afternoons just past, the difficulties were triply compounded.

I've insinuated a couple times that our doctors have provided us little direct help with the swelling legs Kate suffers because of lymphedema. And really, I think this is true, probably because lymphedema results from cancer and is rarely life-threatening. Oncologists are fully committed to eradicating cancer and, therein, potentially saving their patients' lives. Figuring out how to live with the physical and mental side effects of cancer treatment, on the other hand, is largely left to the patient. Certainly medical interaction continues after the immediate crisis of cancer passes. And certainly the transition from a focus on survival to a focus on living is a necessary step for the patient to take. But it can be tough.

Thankfully, one of our Seattle caregivers—perhaps Dr. Cain, Dr. Koh, or their chief nurses Katy or Carol—gave us solid advice for dealing with Kate's lymphedema. They recommended that Kate visit the Northwest Lymphedema Center there in the Seattle area.

The Northwest Lymphedema Center sits on the second floor of a nondescript building in Ballard. A flower store occupies the space below the center; a massage therapist works in the offices next door. Kate first visited the Northwest Lymphedema Center in December 1995, three or four months after returning to work.

Jo Ann Rovig, the center's founder and president, greeted Kate and soon put her through a week of intense study of the lymphatic system. That study helped Kate understand that the removal of lymph nodes for cancer treatment can result in reduced lymph flow and subsequent extremity swelling. Kate also learned Complex Physical Therapy, a method of compression bandaging and massage that helps redirect lymph from occluded or absent passages into those that remain open. The treatment derives from the pioneering work of Australian Drs. John and Judith Casley-Smith and others. Jo Ann also fitted Kate for compression stockings, the same type Kate wears to this day.

At week's end, I joined Kate in Ballard for two days to be trained as a helper in bandaging and massage. By the time we departed, Kate's legs were significantly reduced in size. More important, Jo Ann had provided us with a method to control Kate's lymphedema. Suddenly running and hiking together became possible for us again.

Kate has been lucky not to require nightly compression bandaging, but she wears the stockings daily. We continue to do the massage regularly, and we did so almost every night of our CDT hike.

For us, the Northwest Lymphedema Center was a saving grace. The information and training we received there has significantly improved Kate's quality of life. Yet the center often struggles financially. Although our insurance covered Kate's bills, many insurance companies do not recognize lymphedema as a disease and do not recognize its treatment as a valid medical undertaking. Similarly, some doctors have been slow to accept lymphedema as an important condition. Other doctors are simply unaware that lymphedema can be successfully treated. The people working at the Northwest Lymphedema Center and places like it help their patients overcome the despair of living with a debilitating condition. These good people deserve better.

◪

Back on the Divide, we dropped easily into Goldstone Pass, then climbed steadily toward a cloudless sky. We topped out at 9,731 feet, the highest elevation we'd yet reached on the hike. Open views to the north revealed Homer Youngs Peak and the picket fence of the Bitterroot Range. To the west, smoke and haze hung as the fires of Idaho continued. Eastward, Bloody Dick Creek—named for an Englishman who once lived in the valley—fronted a low range of hills. To the south, the mountains flattened into forested country where the crest of the Divide looked tough to keep track of without a trail.

We took a compass bearing from the map and set out across rocky ridge tops. Only sketchy tread existed at first and we yelled "Blaze!" whenever one of us spotted a notched tree or rock cairn. The trail improved as we dropped into the forest and soon we began a pleasant stroll through the pines. Once a bull elk straddled the trail 30 yards ahead, oblivious to our presence. We watched quietly until some scent or noise or sixth sense warned him. The elk jerked his head upright, stared at us for a brief, wild moment, then raced away at full speed, weaving his large rack through the timber.

Later in the day the blazes and CDT symbols disappeared. After a few dead-end explorations, we opted to follow a jeep track that soon became a high-grade gravel road. Kate and I were pointed toward Pattee Creek, a water source five miles distant. Walking on under intense sun, we started to sag. Kate's legs swelled uncomfortably. The road passed through sullen, industrial forest for mile after mile. Once, we crossed through an active logging operation, quiet for the moment but with hundreds of downed lodgepole pines littered about.

Pattee Creek started as a bit of a disappointment—tiny, little more than a trickle. Its immediate environs included trampled earth and cow pies. Drained and thirsty, Kate dragged herself to the foot-wide dribble and started to pump and purify our evening's water supply. After setting up the tent I relieved her, enjoying the feel of cold water running over my aching feet.

By then a setting sun threw cool crimson light up the drainage. I became immersed in my pumping and was suddenly amazed to see a five-inch trout dart out from under the bank where I sat. Pattee Creek ran six to 18 inches wide there and never more than eight inches deep. Leaning over, I watched the small trout hide under the only available overhang. The fish did not see the swatted horsefly I tossed it, but eight feet downstream another trout rose out of its mossy hiding place and made short work of the offering.

Enthralled and delighted, I looked about and spotted a half dozen other fish from one to six inches long all within ten feet of me, all somehow clinging to life in that threadbare stream. Fifteen feet upstream, Pattee Creek emerged over flat grasses from a tiny spring. The five-inch trout under me was holding in the last possible spot for habitation. To make it this high in the drainage, the fish had crossed a half dozen places where the creek sifted through thick grass covered by little more than an inch of water. In other places, cattle had trampled the channel.

Yet if the odds were stacked against them, if there was ridiculousness in living under these impossible conditions, the trout seemed unaware. Each held strong in its position, facing forward into the current.

◪

Once I asked Kate why, with all the upstream battles—complications, pain, uncertainties—she hadn't at some point just tossed it all in. She didn't feel there was any special magic in her ability to fight through the morass of cancer, but rather just an ongoing willingness to push forward.

For one thing, Kate wasn't willing to just blindly accept her doctors' opinions. "Our doctors suggested that one option was *not* to do anything, to simply accept death as an alternative and optimize the quality of the remainder of my life. When our Portland oncologist told me that, it seemed like part of his job to explain that I could make a choice to do nothing. But when our local doctor—the person I was counting on to help me sort things out—said, "I don't think anyone is talking about a cure here," I felt sick to my stomach. I wanted to say to him, 'How do you know?' I could not accept that as the final answer."

Kate's chemotherapy experience was the lowest of the low times. "The worst I ever felt was during the week of chemo. I was so weak and miserable I would have opted for someone to just shoot me. But once I was all hooked up to everything, barfing my brains out, feeling terrible, there was nothing I could do to escape but wait it out. I was thinking more about getting out of that damn apparatus and all of the vomiting than worrying about surviving cancer."

Later, Kate tackled challenges with a step-by-step approach. "During the middle of the treatment, despite the ups and downs—emergency room visits, surgeries, CAT scans, and so on—I felt like I was working on a project. We had worked out a plan with Dr. Cain and then we implemented it. Mentally, the beginning and end points of treatment were the big adjustments. The middle part, when we were 'working on a project' together, was easier."

Even when she first came home, Kate remembers that the upstream battle did not end. "By the time I got home from the hospital for the last time, I was really worn out. I thought I had gone through all the pain that anyone should have to go through in life and that it was time to start feeling better. But when I ate it hurt so much.

"I thought, 'I can't deal with this pain anymore. I'm worn out. I can't do this anymore.'

"But then I'd lie on the couch, time would pass, I'd get some determination back, go on walks, and things improved."

◤

Cold air hung over Pattee Creek as we packed to move on. The road passed through more industrial, plantation-like forest until Flume Creek, where a sign directed us back onto the Continental Divide Trail. Several sage grouse flushed at our approach shortly after we stepped onto the track. Farther on, four mule deer skittered away through the now wild pines, stopping twenty yards off to eye us curiously, unafraid. The trail followed the ridge through the trees and frequently emerged onto open hillsides covered in bunch grass and sagebrush. When Kate and I stopped on a rock outcropping above Bloody Dick Creek, I spent every moment of the break trying to clear my socks of irritating stickers.

Not long after the break, we rambled over a rise and Lemhi Pass came into view far below us. Suddenly our attention was drawn closer, to where two black figures cut a swath through the sage 50 yards in front of us.

"Look," I whispered to Kate, "black wolves."

Before the words escaped my mouth, I realized the unlikelihood of such a sighting. A second guess that they were two wayward black ranch dogs was also rejected. A moment later, a black bear sow joined her two rollicking cubs. The sow's head rose sufficiently above the sage to leave little doubt of its identity.

The bruins moved slowly across the hillside, from Montana to Idaho, unaware of or unperturbed by our presence. Kate and I watched discreetly, but with admittedly less caution than if the sow and cubs had been grizzly bears.

A few minutes later we slipped down into Montana to give wide berth to the three black bears. We then pushed excitedly on for Lemhi Pass, two miles distant. When we reached the pass, Kate beamed. We slapped hands. This was a major milestone we had dreamed of since back in June, when we had dropped off food at Lemhi Pass on our way to Glacier National Park.

Back then we had looked ahead, thinking, "If we can just make it to Lemhi Pass, 600 miles, then we'll truly have a shot at walking across Montana along the Continental Divide."

At the pass we rejoiced at finding our food still hanging hidden in the forest. And we rejoiced at our progress. Little by little, step-by-step, we were forging ahead. One challenge of long-distance hiking is learning patience, learning to appreciate the process. As with Kate's cancer treatment, we couldn't fully control what might happen the next week, or even the next day. We could only work on what stood in front of us, point ourselves in the right direction, and believe in the ultimate goal.

Kate and I set up the tent at the Sacagawea Memorial Camp, just below the pass, and then looked forward to a much needed rest day. It's interesting that this location was picked to honor Sacagawea, since Lewis chose not to take her along on his first trip over the Divide via this very pass, arguably the most important venture of the Lewis and Clark Expedition. Pushing into unknown country, Lewis hoped to stand on the

Divide and look west into the drainages of the Pacific for the first time. Equally important, he hoped to find friendly Shoshones to provide him with horses, help his Corps of Discovery portage their gear over the Divide, and guide his journey westward.

Sacagawea was a Shoshone, making Lewis's choice to leave her behind during that first foray over Lemhi Pass inexplicable. Instead, Lewis explored the area with just three men and himself. Without Sacagawea as an interpreter, and with little firepower, Lewis was totally unprepared for the Shoshone war party he met on the west side of the Divide. Luckily, Lewis had met a Shoshone woman earlier in the day and plied her with gifts. The woman provided the bridge Lewis and his men needed to gain the Shoshones' confidence.

In the end, the Shoshones provided Lewis with his portage, his horses, and his guide. They also gave him smoked salmon, proof positive to Lewis that he had crossed into the waters of the Columbia. Earlier, Lewis had stopped for a break a short distance below the west side of Lemhi Pass. With possibly more optimism than assurance, he wrote, "here I first tasted the water of the great Columbia river."

A mile away from where Lewis took that first drink, across Lemhi Pass at a tiny spring just beyond our campsite, I was dipping water for the evening meal when a family from California pulled in. Shortly, the kids began noisily producing mud pies. Soon Molly, an adultlike seven year old, brought Kate and me a handwritten menu for the Lewis and Clark Restaurant "runed" by Molly and Sam.

According to the menu, Molly and Sam, her three-year-old brother, were offering "mush" at breakfast . . . and lunch . . . and dinner. Dinner entrees also included "Hambugers" and "Rasberry Chicken." As Kate and I mulled over our selections, their mother Kathy arrived, beers in hand.

"Sorry," Kathy said with a big smile, "I just wanted to come over and apologize for 'The Loud Family.'"

We spent a pleasurable evening and morning in conversation with the Springers. We learned of Kathy's career in paleobiology and her husband Mark's in evolutionary biology (name me another family who would say "glyptodont" instead of "cheese" when mugging for the camera!). Kathy held a bit of California in her soul, addressing her kids as "Sister" and

"Dude." When I commented on Molly's obvious brainpower, suggesting that she might be a budding nuclear scientist, Kathy replied, "Maybe, but I was kind of thinking an actress." For his part, little Sam cranked his Fisher-Price cassette deck, hips gyrating over the picnic table while he yelled, "Rock and roll, *rock and roll!*" Sam had us in stitches.

I tickled the Springer family a bit as well, when I eagerly rescued six stale doughnuts from their garbage bag and promptly devoured them.

I was up before sunrise the morning of our day off. While Kate slept, I climbed halfway back to the Divide, then sat on the cold ground, facing east. Soon, shafts of soft, filtered light dropped onto the Montana hillsides below Lemhi Pass. This was dry, sagebrushy country, desertlike to some, yet I could not imagine a scene more serene or beautiful.

Back at camp, Kate and I eased through the day, reading, resting, and doing restorative couple's yoga. We had learned this form of yoga from a yogi in Corvallis named Sujita, a woman filled with physical and spiritual grace. She had guided us in yoga through the years of Kate's cancer recovery. Sujita helped us recognize the connection between the mind and the body, the power of focusing on the here and now, and the important role that breathing and relaxation play in well-being.

Rejuvenated from the yoga and the day of rest, Kate and I ate a peaceful dinner before I left her to climb to Lemhi Pass to watch the sunset. Out of the ugliness of the fires burning in Idaho emerged an unimaginable beauty. The sun turned smoke hanging over the distant Lemhi Range blood red. Soon the lowering sun scorched the horizon. For a few moments one could see time move, and then the burning ball disappeared.

ELEVEN

Moving On

She says it's long ago, she says it's far away,
she says the past is just a memory.
She says what's gone is gone, she says life still goes on,
she says the times will be what they must be.
The times will be what they must be.

TR RITCHIE
"Changing of the Guard"

THANKS TO A DAY'S REST and lightweight packs—we would pick up food again in only two days—Kate and I rocketed away from Lemhi Pass. It was the end of August. Smoke continued to hang in the western sky, the result of fires still raging in central Idaho. Yet even through the haze, westward views of the Lemhi Range and the Lost River Range inspired us.

Less inspired, one can imagine, was Captain Meriwether Lewis when surveying the same scene. After more than a year's travel through unknown country, his Corps of Discovery stood near this place looking into the Columbia River's upper drainages for the first time. What a disappointment it must have been to see crest after crest of mountain still ahead rather than a simple riverway leading to the Pacific.

Those westerly mountains provided a welcome backdrop as Kate and I made our way up the trail—actually a gravel road at that point—to 9,000 feet. The air was warm, the sun high, and the grass exceedingly short. Cattle and cow pies ruled the ridgeline. Though remote, this was grazing country, country that would be difficult to mistake for wilderness.

Most often the trail followed a fence marking the state boundary. In one Idaho paddock where a hundred cattle milled about, the grass lay dead, brown, and chopped shorter than a putting green. In the adjacent Montana section, which was cow-free, the grasses rose thigh-high except for a barren strip along the fence. Just ahead, as if by way of explanation, a cow strained against the barbwire to reach the tall grass edge.

Kate and I put in nine miles before lunch, a big morning because of the light packs. As we walked on, Goat Mountain came into view, a flat-topped, rocky peninsula jutting out into the Lemhi Valley. The road finally gave out as we approached the flank of the mountain. Grasses grew tall, forest encroached, and the land became less tame. Except for a few sage hens, we had seen no wildlife all morning. But then Kate spotted three mountain goats on Goat Mountain's talus slopes. A moment later I saw seven more, lower and closer, standing in dense brush below the rocks.

We climbed over the notch connecting Goat Mountain to the Divide and then dropped through trailless forest to find a remote camp above the Little Eightmile Valley. I set up the tent while Kate headed out to a rock outcropping to start dinner. Soon I joined her and we quietly absorbed the late afternoon.

Shadows and sunshine accentuated the deep draws and rugged ridge-lines. Goat Mountain's steep, rocky face climbed boldly out of the valley, and its flat top cut the setting sun in half. Far above, just beneath the sun's brilliant halo, two mountain goats crossed the scree.

While we sat waiting for our dinner to cook, I spotted two elk—a four-point bull and a cow—lying in a green patch 250 yards downhill. For 30 minutes the elk rested peacefully, then suddenly they stood up and looked about in a panic. Quickly the elk focused their anxieties uphill, and in another instant they bolted into the trees.

It was a full minute before Kate and I heard the drone of two OHVs. By the time the OHVs bounced down one side of the valley and roared up to where we sat, four or five minutes had passed since the elk had exited. The OHV riders had bows and quivers strapped to their big-wheeled machines. Both men wore camouflage. As the men came over a slight rise, their faces showed considerable surprise at seeing us.

"Where'd *you* come from?" they asked after turning their machines off. I explained about the CDT walk as both men lit cigarettes.

As I wound down my story, one of them looked out over his OHV's handlebars and asked, "So y'all seen any elk?"

September 1, 1998. We awoke next to Goat Mountain, muscles eager for the day. After hot tea, we pulled on the packs and started walking toward the cool morning sunrise. Quickly we saw a lone elk at forest's edge and I suddenly felt overwhelmed with joy—can there be any greater, simpler pleasure than carrying one's own gear through the mountains?

Hiking over a small ridge, Kate and I came fully into the remote upper valley of Little Eightmile Creek. The valley cut first across a high, wide plateau, then wedged through a slot in the mountains on its way to the Lemhi River. Though cattle abounded there, the expansive country still breathed with seclusion. We walked along the treeless state boundary, passing a couple of hunters' camps before sliding back into forest when the fence line gave out. Some easy compass work got us across wooded Grizzly Hill. Though we had seen no CDT symbols for miles, as soon as the fence line returned, we marched ahead with confidence.

After Grizzly Hill the country went flat and the trail soon crossed open, sagebrush plains. It was a bit of a stretch to believe that we were walking on the crest of the continent. The sun grew hot as the land grew parched. With each step we kicked up a fine dust that hung in the air.

Near Bannock Pass we recovered the food we had left a month earlier in one of the area's few trees. The gravel road crossing the Divide stood quiet; no vehicles passed during the half hour we sorted through our rations. Finishing up, Kate sheepishly asked what I might think of hitching into Leadore, Idaho, 12 miles west, for an unplanned shower. With two weeks of grime already built up and another week before our next expected shower, the idea sounded as delectable as it did preposterous, given the lack of traffic. But fifteen minutes on, saints be praised, we saw the distant dust plume of a vehicle heading up the pass from Horse Prairie Creek.

An hour later, as if by magic, Kate and I sat back on a soft bed, showered and clean, our remaining clothes in the wash at Leadore's only motel. A shower after weeks of sweat and dust may be the ultimate feel-good experience. Only an unexpected shower in the same circumstance is better.

In the morning, we found most of Leadore's population gathered at the café near the motel. Everyone wanted in—pickups crowded the small parking lot and even a small plane sat tail-in to the building. Kate and I slipped quietly into seats at the remaining table, but even in our beat-up duds we clearly stood out. When I asked for the largest stack of pancakes the cook could make, somebody at the counter said, "You two must be hikers."

Following breakfast, we headed to the post office, where Lisa Martini, the postmaster, informed us that a number of Continental Divide Trail hikers had already stopped in that year. She pulled out the CDT log for us, which revealed that folks we'd met on the trail—Nick, Dan and Sara, and David and Andrew—had all been through in late July or early August. David wrote that he could never get enough food and that he and Andrew had seen a hundred elk below Goat Mountain. Dan and Sara worried about the weight of the eight days' food they would require to reach Mack's Inn. One theme common to everyone was that the trail in southwest Montana was poorly marked.

Someone had written in the logbook pretending to be Lewis and Clark:

> After years and years (almost 2 centuries) we have still not reached the conclusion of our journey for President Jefferson. Our Corps of Discovery was almost out of provisions when we discovered this tiny settlement. Still seeking the return route east to St. Louis on this confusing damn trail (CDT).
>
> Captains Lewis and Clark
>
> P.S. Who removed all those markers we put up?

In a note written in remarkably similar handwriting to that of Lewis and Clark, Nick Williams called the CDT the "Connect-The-Dots" trail and mentioned hiking with "my good friend JoAnne." JoAnne was a hiker Kate and I had never met, but someone we had heard about along the trail. Back near Rogers Pass we'd told Nick, who was hiking alone, to keep an eye out for her. In our ample dreaming time, Kate and I had concocted a story as we walked that Nick and the unknown JoAnne would meet and become a couple. Here now was startling proof; the CDT—a sweaty, blistering soap opera!*

Other log entries pulled us deeper into the brotherhood of the trail. Notes from years past included one from Walkin' Jim Stoltz and one from the McVeighs, the couple who had made a video ("Journey on the Continental Divide") of their trip along the Divide. Jim Wolf, the author of our hiking guide, had been through this year as had Fiddlehead, a hiker David had told us about. Fiddlehead wrote about getting stronger. Shortly before arriving in Leadore, Fiddlehead had walked one evening into the dark, totaling 29 miles for the day and feeling he could have done more.

Twenty-nine miles sounded like a heck of a day's hike to Kate and me. Our longest walk of the trip had just touched 16 miles.

How far can people really go in a day? Gear Nazi Ray Jardine, the lightweight hiking aficionado, writes of walking *39 consecutive days averaging 33.9 miles per day* along the Pacific Crest Trail. Bob Marshall, forester and cofounder of the Wilderness Society, claimed regular day hikes of 40 miles. In his biography of Marshall, *A Wilderness Original: The Life of Bob Marshall*, James Glover writes that Marshall held such a passion for the four-decade milestone that "he was known to go out after supper on a Sunday night to walk up and down the road if he needed another mile or two to make it an even 40 for the day."

Kate and I added our thoughts, which made no proud claim to daily mileages hiked, to the CDT logbook. Almost two years after our stop in Leadore, postmaster Martini graciously sent me a copy of our logbook entry, which ended:

> . . . *And so it's been a blessed journey for us. A time of peace, simplicity, serenity. A time to celebrate turning away cancer. During the planning stages of this trip a friend gave us a card that said, "All great things begin with a dream." Now with West Yellowstone and the end of this segment of our lives just weeks away, we can only think to add, " . . . and all great things must end with a little bit of sadness."*

*In a delightful footnote to the story, Nick and JoAnne recently married!

Before cancer, Kate and I too often had to steal time from our busy schedules to be alone, to pursue our dreams, to allow ourselves the time to turn inward. Cancer helped us recognize that sad state of affairs. What could possibly be a more important demand of our time than fighting to regain Kate's health?

During Kate's struggle to get well, we drastically dropped our participation in activist organizations and cut back on our appointments. We stopped booking 150 percent of our time. We let go of petty aggravations and things we could not control. We said "no" to friends and family when we needed to, and we learned to accept the discomfort that that action brought. We began to say "yes" only to those things most precious to us. With cancer we suddenly had a rallying point to judge all activities against.

Being "selfish" became important to Kate's healing process because it helped us control our lives instead of being swept along by schedules run amok. To most people, the idea of focusing on themselves feels egotistical, vain, or misanthropic. Many people thus pursue a distinctly "selfless" approach to life, one in which they spend little time nourishing their own spirits. While a selfless lifestyle may be sustainable in regular life, for Kate, fighting cancer mandated a turn inward.

Kate learned early in our cancer experience that to give her body and mind their best chance at healing, she had to declare a space of her own. Everyone around her—friends and family, neighbors and workmates—wanted nothing more than to help. Perhaps the considerate thing for Kate to do would have been to welcome others' expressions of pain without condition. But while an outpouring of heartfelt grief—or even hysteria—might have made the giver feel better, it would have done little to help Kate and might, in fact, have set her back a step. Shared love is a wonderful positive, but others' raw grief had the power to smother Kate. We avoided those confrontations whenever possible.

Once, while in the hospital, Kate declared that she was not willing to be part of somebody else's tragedy. "Part of my need for privacy," Kate says now, "was that I didn't want to spread the painfulness to other people. And part of it was that I didn't want to expose my pain to everyone else. I didn't want cancer to be the primary topic that everyone would talk to me about."

Kate had difficulty maintaining her identity. "It kind of reinforces the tragedy and disability of the disease when that's all anyone talks about. It's like you become the disease. Perhaps for me seeking privacy was a combined form of denial and survival."

Friends and family were (and are) critically important to Kate's healing progress, absolutely, but so was (and is) time spent alone. Kate often needed to be selfish to survive. Others might find cancer a reason to turn outward, to seek solace from friends, loved ones, or a support group. No right answer exists. There are as many ways to cope with the stress of a life-threatening disease as there are people.

◤

Around noon the next day, the motel proprietor kindly shuttled us from Leadore back to Bannock Pass. The climb away from the pass proved to be long, hot, and empty. Kate and I followed barbwire for six miles, over Deadman Pass and then up to the edge of the trees and the start of the big climbs.

As we ate lunch, we looked back over the golden, treeless expanse of Bannock Pass country. In the early 1900s a railroad company built a line across the pass. The hoped-for commerce, however, never arrived. The line failed, as one historian wrote, because the railroad "started from nowhere, traversed through nothing, and ended up nowhere."

With all that emptiness, little anchored Kate and me in our own time. One could easily imagine a distant dust cloud, far out on Horse Prairie Creek, signaling the approach of Chief Joseph and his struggling band of Nez Percé. Back in 1877, after the Nez Percé had defeated the U.S. Army in the Battle of the Big Hole, the Indians struck out to the south. The Nez Percé paralleled the east face of the Continental Divide—just below where Kate and I had been walking during the past two weeks—before eventually descending Bloody Dick Creek to Horse Prairie. The army pursued, their charge of moving the Indians onto an Idaho reservation unchanged even after the defeat at the Big Hole. The Nez Percé ascended

Horse Prairie Creek and then crossed Bannock Pass just below where we now sat. The legendary flight of the Nez Percé would go from Bannock Pass, along the south side of the Centennials, through the newly founded Yellowstone Park, then north to the Missouri River.

In the end, General Howard would stop the bedraggled Nez Percé 1,700 miles after their flight began, in the Bear Paw Mountains just 42 miles from the safety of Canada. It was there in October of 1877 that Chief Joseph, a man revered for his leadership, compassion, and military acumen, uttered these famous lines to his captors:

> I am tired of fighting. Our chiefs are killed. Looking Glass is dead. The old men are all killed. It is the young men who say yes or no. He who led the young men is dead. It is cold and we have no blankets. The little children are freezing to death. My people, some of them, have run away to the hills and have no blankets, no food; no one knows where they are, perhaps freezing to death. I want time to look for my children and see how many of them I can find. Maybe I shall find them among the dead. Hear me, my chiefs, I am tired; my heart is sick and sad. From where the sun now stands, I will fight no more forever.

Kate and I finished lunch and then turned away from the imagined Nez Percé. We climbed steeply from the tawny grasslands through thin forest and then out onto the tussock* above tree line. An unnamed 10,000-foot peak loomed ahead. Just beyond that a slightly higher summit, Elk Mountain, pushed into the cloudless sky. A gentle wind, warm even at that altitude, guided us upward. Chocolate brown, burnt orange, and fiery yellow alpine grasses contrasted vividly with the steel gray talus of the summits. We walked on and up, as if into a painting.

Elk Mountain's 10,194-foot summit was the highest point we would reach along the Montana Divide. Kate and I topped out easily, six and a half hours after leaving Bannock Pass. A metal spike, the Divide marker, rose from a rock pile at the summit. Ahead, the highest mountains along Montana's Divide, 11,000-plus-foot Cottonwood and Eighteenmile

*A landscape characterized by compact tufts of grass.

Peaks, showed through the haze. Closer at hand the Divide seemed less obvious, with a funny hitch in it near Tepee Mountain that we could not decipher.

No clouds threatened, so we pulled out our sleeping pads and sat contemplatively for most of an hour. Even with two longish stops, we had put in ten miles in little over five hours—not bad for us considering our food-heavy packs and the 2,700-foot elevation gain. Kate and I talked about how strong we felt, and how thankful we were that the trail had tempered us, not shattered us.

A cooling breeze chased us off Elk Mountain. We dropped steeply through loose scree and big boulders. Paint marks and rock cairns showed periodically, allowing us to concentrate on negotiating the rubble rather than searching for the trail. Soon we found new tread and even a CDT reassurance symbol. Once we were off the summit and back below the tree line, Kate and I followed a suggestion from Wolf and camped near Reservoir Creek.

Because of our late morning start, dinner lasted into darkness. After the dishes were washed, Kate and I walked to the forest's edge to hang our food. The deep shadows ended there—the field before us glowed in the soft light of a rising moon.

I walked back out to the field early the next morning, wanting to see the sun rise. Instead I found myself immersed in smoke. It felt like I was wading through dense fog, but with an added bitter smell and no cooling sensation. When the sun finally peeked over the horizon, it emerged as a distant pumpkin, muted orange and eerie.

Back at the tent, Kate said she thought she had smelled smoke settling during the night. At 2 A.M. the distant bugle of an elk had awakened me. I hadn't slept much after that, sniffling with what I thought were allergies. Likely it was the smoke.

In Leadore we had watched the news and learned that much of the smoke we had been seeing on and off since Chief Joseph Pass had been coming from Idaho's River of No Return Wilderness. Fourteen fires, amalgamated as the "Main Salmon Complex," were expected to burn into the fall. West winds pushed the fires' smoke to the Divide where it sometimes became trapped, as on this day.

By the time Kate and I walked away from camp the sun burned stronger, but the smoke washed out even the nearby hillsides. We could no longer see the distant Red Conglomerate Peaks nor, much closer at hand, towering Baldy Mountain. In the end we would have to walk half of the ten miles toward Baldy Mountain before we could even distinguish its outline.

We pushed ahead, walking for hours as though through an endless smoky barroom. By noon, despite the smoke, the sun blazed down. I sweated profusely as the humidity ran surprisingly high for such dry country. We climbed a jeep road through open, smoky benchlands to cross three 9,500-foot rises, all without the benefit of shade. Finally we dropped off the benchlands, then rolled over a couple of final knolls to beautiful, desolate Morrison Lake.

Kate wasted little time in submersing herself in the cold waters. I followed shortly. We did yoga as our dinner simmered, thankful for the cooling air and dissipating smoke.

In the morning we followed rock cairns and CDT posts past Simpson and Tex Creeks. The country there—mostly deep, narrow canyons spilling out into a flat basin—was ruggedly beautiful and heavily grazed. Atop the Coyote Creek drainage we stopped for lunch before climbing onto a magical plateau: an endless alpine meadow devoid of tree or shrub, filled with red and yellow and amber and orange grasses. Cottonwood Peak stood darkly behind, a massive earth wall with valleys and ridges that rolled off it like waves.

The tawny coats of five antelope provided a mild contrast to the lustrous grasses. Already that morning, back near Morrison Lake, we had seen 45 antelope out on the plains. Like those, these five eyed us warily. As we continued to walk, the antelope took flight, crossing the highest slope of a 9,700-foot peak. We had never seen antelope so high on a mountain, but then why not? Like the plains they usually inhabit, no trees, indeed nothing, interrupted their ability to spot predators in that dreamy landscape.

Knowing that we wanted to end up on the side of Cottonwood Peak, but uncertain how best to get there, I consulted our guidebooks. One of them said that a rock cairn sitting on a knoll would mark the correct route. I pointed myself toward a potential mound, but Kate thought otherwise. As we began to separate, I yelled to her, "I'm going with the guidebook."

Kate called back, "I'm going with the antelope."

Kate and the antelope found the next trail marker long before I did. While she rounded the head of Meadow Creek, I dropped into the drainage and then climbed out onto the flank of Cottonwood Peak. I rejoined Kate at about 9,000 feet and then we climbed through deep, steep grasslands to around 9,800 feet at the Divide. Two antelope yo-yoed up the mountain with us, waiting until we approached to within 50 yards of them, then skipping ahead again.

Atop the Divide came more austere beauty: the ochre grasslands of Big Sheep Creek to the east, the imposing skyline of the Lemhi Range to west, and before us the swelling shoulder of Cottonwood Peak. In every direction the land opened itself to the sky. We looked down from the top of the world, alone but for two friendly antelope. Kate and I sat for a time, sweat drying, heart rates dropping, until a dark cloud drove us off the ridgeline. Hail spit down for a brief time, then beams of sun chased the darkness away.

Down the east slopes of Cottonwood Peak we found a two-foot-wide creek running clear and fast. Kate slipped her bare feet into the icy water, then squealed in pain and delight. We camped embarrassingly close to the little creek on the only flat ground available—the only plot of ground not covered with sagebrush and stickers. The creek curled around the tent so tightly that all night we drifted on the sound of its waters, at peace as the world raced by.

◼

A spouse, a friend, or a family member can play a critical role in helping a cancer patient—the role of an advocate. An advocate is a person who provides love, support, and understanding. An advocate assists with daily tasks and helps the patient's life keep moving. I cannot imagine how difficult it must be to tackle a debilitating disease alone.

As Kate's advocate I could act as her interface: assuring friends that we still existed, sharing her status, and encouraging visitors when the time was right. I could also help maintain Kate's desire for privacy by shielding her from well-meaning friends during the worst of times.

Kate told me, "I think that if you had not run interference for me, I would have been too closed off on my own. I wouldn't have received all of the support, calls, visits, cards, flowers, and good wishes if it hadn't been for you informing people of what was going on. I felt that a lot of people cared about me in a way that they are afraid to show in ordinary circumstances."

Even amid the bedlam of the cancer, I was thankful that I could keep us moving forward as a couple, as a team.

The advocate's role can go deeper, too, to keeping track of medical visits and researching the available treatments. The pain of learning of her disease, and later of dealing with the treatments, left Kate little stamina. "I would not have had the energy to do the research that you did," she told me. "It helped me early on to hear you say 'Look, here's a case where this person was worse off than you, and they were completely healed by such and such treatment.'

"Knowing that there could be a thread of hope," she continued, "really made a difference. Also, because of your research you were able to ask the doctors really good questions, and they were able to adjust or defend their approaches. Asking that one extra question or tracking bits of data can bring out valuable discussion and sometimes change the course of the treatment plan."

We were fortunate that I could spend every moment of Kate's healing process with her. Some folks, we realize, are not so lucky. Kate said, "I think that having you as my primary caregiver at home and in the hospital was much more intimate and supportive than any other alternative could have been."

We feel humbly blessed that I could undertake such a strong advocate's position. Yet less all-consuming work can certainly be critical as well—for example, marshaling friends, taking care of the bills, managing the house, and shopping for groceries. It's important that an advocate's efforts allow the patient time to concentrate on healing. Most important, I think, is that an advocate acts out of love.

◤

After climbing over a ridge to Rock Creek, the CDT drops far away from Cottonwood Peak and the Divide. The trail slips down through whitebark pine forest to the open valley floor, then passes desolate Harkness Lakes before rolling pleasantly through sagebrush to crossings of Bear, Tendoy, and Nicholia Creeks. The Divide proper quickly forms a distant southerly backdrop as the trail short-circuits Montana's southernmost protrusion.

Following that route, Kate and I found ourselves eating lunch along Nicholia Creek the day following our camp on the side of Cottonwood Peak. The walking had been easy and the temperatures cool, but Kate had been dragging. She worried out loud that her body was telling her something and then declared that she had better listen. We decided to forgo our original goal for the day of Deadman Lake, five miles on.

We found a pleasant camp shortly up the valley on a bench above Nicholia Creek. Dense willows blanketed the broad valley floor. Ahead, heavily wooded sidehills climbed into rugged mountains. Soon we had the tent up. Kate climbed inside to read and nap while I prepared to go fishing.

Sixty yards away, a large bull moose appeared in the creek bottom. This was a substantial animal with a colossal rack. Seeing me, the moose moved deeper into the willows, though he looked more put out than afraid. Later, after I went fishing, pounding hooves woke Kate. She slowly unzipped the tent. The big bull stood 20 yards away on the edge of the willows, staring at her. Kate stared back. The standoff ended when Kate zipped up the tent so that she could return to her sleep, but the moose's munching kept her awake for an hour. When I returned from fishing, the moose glared at me, then moved slowly away again.

Shortly, Kate and I walked downstream around a distant bend in the creek to prepare dinner. As we cooked, the moose reappeared, now perhaps 200 yards away. He walked and browsed in the willows, walked and browsed, always moving in our direction. Soon he was 50, then 40 yards away.

The moose stopped browsing then and walked out of the willows directly toward us, glaring at us. I looked back and told Kate that we would crawl under an enormous downed spruce if the moose kept coming. Thirty yards, twenty. We sat poised for retreat.

The moose stopped at the creek's edge, still glowering, then lowered his head, shaking his massive rack. Next he bared his teeth and groaned, almost growled. We took that as our cue to move back to the protective tree. For ten minutes we watched this absurdly large animal watch us. All the while steam rose from our neglected pasta dish. Finally the moose begrudgingly moved off.

From my journal that night:

> *As I write this, in the sleeping bag, an owl calls. Kate claims she can hear the moose chomping somewhere out in the willows. I search back in my mind, trying to recall if I've ever read about anyone being attacked in their tent by a moose.*

In the morning another bull moose, smaller and less certain of itself, trotted down Nicholia Creek toward us through wet willows and low fog. At a hundred yards the moose scented us and stopped. Steam blew from his nostrils, leaving his face in a cloud. The moose watched us for fully 15 minutes as we packed. Then he suddenly cut the distance in half, approaching aggressively before stopping and turning broadside. Kate and I decided that the breeding season must be underway and that the rut was driving the bull moose crazy. When we shouldered our packs, the moose trotted away up the other side of the valley. He was at once gangly and graceful.

Kate and I followed the moose up the creek a short distance before climbing out of the Nicholia Basin. The Divide proper sidles around the parallel drainages of Nicholia and Deadman Creeks. The CDT, however, crosses between the two streams several miles below the Divide. We followed the trail over the ridge, through Henderson Gulch, and then down into Deadman Lake, which sits in a deep cleft between the mountains. The trail merged with a jeep road before plunging down to the lake. The road fell away at such a precipitous angle as to make for uncomfortable hiking, much less driving.

Though we had quit early the previous day, Kate and I decided more rest was in order, so we pulled up at Deadman Lake after hiking only five miles. Across the lake, three fishermen plunked worms unsuccessfully. Later five more motored in, then nine horsemen arrived, then five OHVers showed up. Here in this little-known corner of Montana we saw more people than anywhere in the state outside of Glacier Park. When someone reminded us it was Labor Day weekend, the crowds made a bit more sense.

By early evening, Kate and I were alone at the lake, save for a cow moose and two beavers that had emerged to patrol their domain. Kate felt rejuvenated after a second half day of resting through the afternoon. I felt giddy. I had fished all day with stunning success to wild cutthroats that slashed at small dry flies—one after another, beautiful, deeply colored fish.

When dusk settled, bats emerged to wing silently over the lake, challenging hungry trout for hovering mayflies. On into twilight the fish rose until finally, overwhelmed, I paused from casting to yell at Kate, "I am having *way* more fun here than could possibly be legal."

"That's all right," she replied, her headlamp flashing as she looked up from her book, "you deserve it."

What I—what we—might or might not deserve I didn't know. I did know that each and every day I was looking forward to the next, excited for whatever new challenge awaited, excited for what we would see, excited for sunrise and breakfast and packing to move ahead.

I also knew that every day we were cutting a substantial chunk out of the 200 miles remaining between Lemhi Pass and Yellowstone Park. Suddenly the hike had started to grow edges and it saddened me. This life was rich and substantial; we yearned for the day to be long, for more time to experience all that was available. Our minds were clear, our bodies radiated fitness, and our souls soared above us.

◢

October 1996. It was almost four years after the original cancer diagnosis but still several months before we began serious preparations for hiking Montana's Continental Divide. Kate sat in tall grass near the tent, knitting. That morning we had backpacked up a desert canyon along our favorite eastern Oregon stream. Fall colors tipped the willows. Crisp air and clear skies foretold an icy night.

Kate's stomach had been troubling her, and her legs were swollen. Thus she had stayed at the tent while I headed upstream to fish.

"Cuppa tea?" I asked upon my return to camp.

Kate looked up, her eyes filled with tears. Ignoring my question she said quietly, "It's been two years today since my surgery. The doctor said I had a one in ten chance of living until now."

Every single day I marvel at how Kate can march ahead with the tasks at hand, even when struggling with the memories of what cancer has taken from her and with all the problems cancer treatment has brought to her life. I've seen her cry many times, at home and on the trail, in anger or in sadness. Yet countless times I've also seen her snap quickly back, unwilling to let sadness overcome her. I often wonder if I would have the same courage. "How do you cope so readily?" I asked one day.

"Sure, I get mad at my lymphedema, bladder infections, and bowel problems," she replied, "but I accept them as part of the cost of getting to live. I really get mad that my legs swell. I wear pants or try not to look at them. I swear to myself I'll do a lymphedema massage and get the swelling down overnight. I get really frustrated when I think about them, so I try not to spend much time thinking about them."

"But how do you keep moving forward," I asked, "rather than stalling right there and dropping off into the doldrums?"

Her answer was simple: "Usually we're doing something way more fun than thinking about what hurts, so I just keep doing what we're doing and I think to myself, 'Look, I can still do this.'"

"We live on happily," I wrote in my journal shortly after the last of Kate's cancer treatments, "because we are thankful, and to live sadly would be useless. Having cancer is like being an alcoholic. It will be something we always think of, that we can't run from or escape from, that will become entwined in the fabric of our lives. May we somehow turn cancer into a golden thread."

◪

For the second day running, Kate and I woke to bugling elk. We broke camp, then climbed from Deadman Lake back to the Divide, a crisp wind buffeting us the entire way. Heavy cumulus clouds bounced across the sky. The clouds seemed to portend some change of weather. Yet as we moved along, rain threatened but never appeared. We comforted ourselves with the thought that most storms must surely bypass these vast, dry grasslands.

Kate and I spilled off the ridgelines out onto the high plains and treeless expanse of Medicine Lodge Pass. The Blackfeet Indians are reputed to have built a medicine lodge near that spot for performing rituals to protect themselves in battle. The lodge likely appeared as a gargantuan tepee covered in buffalo robes. The structure focused inward to its most sacred element, a giant center pole.

The ceremonies carried out in the medicine lodge sometimes included severe self-torture practiced by young warriors. In a 1947 narrative, Blood Indian Heavy, one of the last Blackfeet to undergo this painful ordeal, described his experience. Blood Indian Heavy wore only a breechcloth. Three old men of the tribe painted his entire body, including four black dots under each of his eyes. These dots were called "tear paint" and would show his tears. Then another Indian, Red Bead, approached with a sharp, iron arrowhead. As Blood Indian Heavy related:

> . . . he pierced my breasts with the sharp arrowhead and inserted a sarvis berry stick through each breast. These sticks were not sharp but flattened at the ends. Blood flowed down my chest and legs over the white paint. . . .
>
> Rawhide ropes were brought out from the center pole and tied to skewers in my breast—right side first, then left side. Red Bead grabbed the ropes and jerked them hard twice. Then he told me, "Now go to the center pole and pray for your vow to come true." I walked up there. I knew I was supposed to pretend to cry. But oh! I really cried. It hurt so

much. Coming back from the center pole, I was shouting. . . .

I leaned back and began dancing, facing the center pole. It felt like the pole was pulling me toward it. I danced from the west toward the doorway of the lodge and back. Then, when the skewers didn't break loose, the old men realized that the incisions had been made too deep. Red Bead cut the outside of the incisions so they would break loose. As I started dancing again the left side gave way and I continued dancing with only my right side holding. Then an old man, Strangling Wolf, got up from the crowd and called out four war honors, then jumped upon me. The second rope gave way and I fell to the ground.

The three old men cut off the rough pieces of flesh hanging from my breasts. They told me to take these trimmings and the sagebrush from my wrists, ankles, and head and place them at the base of the center pole as my offering to the sun. . . .

In the midst of the quiet and peace around us, Kate and I found it impossible to imagine the excruciating pain that the warriors suffered through. Looking about, we saw no signs of the medicine lodge. Instead, while standing by a gate we had just crossed, we saw an approaching horseman, so we waited and held the gate open for him.

The horseman, John Morgan, was a bow-toting elk hunter from Idaho Falls. We had met plenty of hunters in the past week: a couple of spry octogenarian grouse hunters from Butte, ten grouse-hunting friends beating the brush with an equal number of dogs, numerous pre-season bow hunters scouting for elk, and two well-prepared Divide hunters from the East Coast—they'd purchased elk tags for Montana *and* Idaho.

John wore camouflage army pants and a tan Stetson. His face carried smudges of green paint. On the way in to hunt, John told us, his packhorse had shied at the gate and fought him hard before going through. John's saddle horse, Gunner, was a bit skittish as well.

"Don't know why," John said holding a tight rein. "Sure ain't like he don't get rode much."

John and his two-horse team passed through the gate without incident. As I rehooked the fence, John thanked us and then asked us to join him for a soda at his truck. By the time we met him there 15 minutes later, the offer turned into an invitation to lunch.

John, a considerably slim guy, said, "My wife always tells me, 'You never eat when you're elk hunting.' Look at all this food she sent with me. You two can help make it look like I ate a bit more. Here, how about a turkey sandwich?"

My wife ate with unabashed gluttony. Kate wolfed her way into a monstrous sandwich while drinking a cola, the second she'd accepted from a hunter in a week, and the first two in modern memory.

The hike had definitely stamped its imprint on Kate's hunger. Each of the previous two days she had asked me to supplement our food supply with trout. Although usually squeamish around fish, Kate peeled away the bones and dug in without reserve. She had even asked me to try and buy food from some of the fisherman we had seen at Deadman Lake.

Walking down the rutted road an hour before meeting John, Kate had spied and then *pounced* on a box of raisins sitting in the dirt. "My God," she cried, "food from heaven!" She poured half the raisins into her hand, then handed the box to me.

"You're actually going to eat those raisins?" I asked in disbelief. This is a woman who normally won't drink a cup of tea stirred with someone else's spoon.

"I think they're all right," Kate replied. She greedily popped the raisins into her mouth and then, talking as she chewed, said, "It's so dry here. Besides, they probably just got dropped by those OHVers from yesterday."

I poured the remaining raisins into my hand. Six ants came out of the box with the raisins. Flicking the ants away, I swallowed the raisins in a single mouthful. Now an hour later, there with John, I had yet to tell Kate of my observation.

While we ate, John talked of bow hunting. "Year-round," John said fervently. "I love bow huntin'. Don't fish much anymore."

John's T-shirt showed that he had won an off-season archery competition. When talk turned to calling in the elk, John's enthusiasm didn't drop a notch. "Out huntin' sometimes you just play with the bulls, buglin' back and forth at each other. It's so much fun. I just love bein' out here whether I shoot one of them bad boys or not. Haven't got one in three years. But this year we need the meat."

John paused to push some Pop-Tarts our way. Then his face beamed. "Calling them in is so incredible. I got one to come in on me when I was hidin' out in the sagebrush. That bad boy came a snortin' and a huffin' out of the trees, ready to tear me apart. He got 30 yards from me. You have to sit there *so* still. Tough part is drawin' back the arrow without spookin' 'em. Man, that bull was ready to kill somethin'. I drew back just as he figured out what I was. That's when I dropped that bad boy."

As John closed his story, he reached back into his food box for more goodies. By now Kate had finished her sandwich and was starting into the lunch we'd brought for ourselves. Looking up to see John reaching out with an offering, Kate said, "What? A granola bar? Sure, John, thanks a lot."

◹

Backpacking is a lot like life. Beyond a certain point, the more "stuff" you carry with you, the harder it is to progress.

Cancer has taught Kate and me one thing if nothing else: *Simplicity breeds well-being.* We've come to realize that we cannot do everything and be everything to everyone and still have time to be ourselves. And we've learned that carrying around too much stuff—be it the mental garbage of a poor relationship or the physical garbage of an over-consumptive lifestyle—is simply unhealthy. In every way, Western society seems pro-grammed to drive us to more, more, more. Learning when to say, "Enough!" has become important to our well-being.

The new focus has brought us tangible changes: greater closeness with each other, more time to read, fewer work hours, and less stress. And coincident with our commitment to simplicity has come a new definition of success. Though we had never been tightly tied into the great American dream, cancer turned our focus even farther away from main-stream goals. Today we value most strongly substantive relationships and causes that are core to our essence. We value, more deeply than ever, con-necting with people and—if we are able—helping them.

It's odd how simple changes like those I've just mentioned can seem revolutionary. So often Kate and I have heard, "Wow, I bet cancer has really changed your definition of what's important. I bet it's been a real wake-up call."

Well yes . . . and no. Cancer has modified our outlook on life, sure. But we have not done an about-face in our belief systems, approach to life, or relationships with friends. Kate and I often thought of ourselves as people who were already pursuing our dreams, who didn't need a "wake-up call" to start experiencing life. Indeed, memories of our life experiences often helped us cope with the thought that death waited just over the next rise.

TR Ritchie once wrote:

> *You have to make yourself let go of broken dreams*
> *before you can believe in any other kind.*

I think that's the greatest mental change cancer has brought to us: a loss of innocence. Once Kate and I had dreams that seemed boundless. Now we recognize limits. In truth it's simply been a change in outlook, not a change in reality. Some might call it "growing up." Indeed, cancer is not a prerequisite for such a realization.

It's true that some of our dreams have disappeared since the cancer. *Lost* dreams, however, do not equate to *no* dreams. Once Kate told me she would rather die than lose her ability to dream. A critical part of Kate's healing has been her ability—if not downright dogged resolve—to make room for new dreams, and to look ahead.

◢

By the time John Morgan climbed into his rig and headed toward Idaho, Kate and I had hiked half the distance from Medicine Lodge Pass to the white carbonate cliffs far above. Kate raced along as though she had been shot out of a cannon. She claimed to be levitating on calories and caffeine. I followed as she floated above the ground, past the cliffs and then up onto an endless grassy plateau.

Walking through vast country, wind whistling, we suddenly became aware of a vehicle behind us, an unusual feeling in such an empty place. As the pickup pulled alongside, the driver waved. Mark Anderson, we soon learned, worked for the Montana Department of Fish, Wildlife, and Parks. Mark wore a ball cap and chewed tobacco. He was checking on hunters and looking for OHV riders gone bad. He expressed anger as we told him of the OHVers we'd seen at Deadman Lake. Mark said they had illegally crossed vast closed areas. But he didn't express a lot of hope in catching them.

"We just don't have enough manpower. I'm the only enforcement officer that patrols this area, and I live 60 miles away in Dillon."

As Mark talked, I peered into the cab. The dashboard contained all manner of electronic equipment. A spotting scope sat on the seat; a rifle was mounted to the ceiling. When Mark paused to turn down the static on one of his radios, I changed topics, asking him about grizzly bear sightings. Though still almost a hundred miles from Yellowstone Park, only I-15 and a lot of wild country separated us from there.

"I hear lots of grizzly reports every year," Mark replied, adjusting the tobacco wad with his tongue. "Some you toss out immediately, some you can't be sure of, and some are *real* interesting. We've had a couple reports not far from here in the Muddy Creek drainage that I'm intrigued by. The bottom line, though, is nothing has been substantiated. You know there's a lot of dimorphism in these black bears. Some people see the blonde color and that's it—it's a grizzly. They're tough to convince otherwise."

Mark's road headed uphill while the CDT posts began a sidehill traverse. Kate stopped for a moment after Mark departed, but I continued on, walking through tall grasses from post to post since no trail existed. Once a coyote bolted out of the grass in front of me, but mostly the land breathed only with the wind. And the land was awesome: endless, tawny grasslands cascaded off to the north, falling away to Big Sheep Creek, which sliced a green swath through dry country. Beyond the valley, spur ridges and deep ravines rose up to the high hills of the Tendoy Mountains. Behind us Baldy, Cottonwood, and Eighteen Mile peaks stretched for the sky. Directly ahead a massive pyramid of rock, 10,961-foot Garfield Mountain, dominated the countryside. Garfield Mountain sat purple in the shade of distant storm clouds.

With grass and canyon, hill and valley, sun and clouds, it was all too big and open and empty to absorb. I stopped and tried, overwhelmed by the enormity of it all, then looked back to see Kate making her way gamely through the tall grass. Out of nowhere my mind flashed to her hospital bed almost four years earlier. I saw Kate bloated by the combination of chemotherapy and 20 pounds of IV fluids, Kate retching at the smell of food. A lump grew large in my throat as Kate came nearer. She plopped down and, as so often happens, our minds were one. Without a question to me, without looking at me, without having discussed cancer in days or maybe even a week, she said, "Do you remember how in the hospital we used to talk them into unhooking me, so we could go outside to breathe the fresh air? We'd just stand there in the sun and breathe. Breathe in now." She filled her lungs. "Isn't it wonderful?"

An hour later Kate and I stopped for the night near a grove of aspens, a few of which showed hints of yellowing. After putting up the tent, we climbed onto a saddle to cook. The imposing façade of Garfield Mountain commanded the scene, separated from us only by the valley of Little Sheep Creek. Dense purple clouds moved hard and fast overhead. Shining sheets of rain showed under holes in the clouds, but the droplets did not reach the ground. Shafts of low-angle sun hopscotched across the scene, and then a rainbow formed a perfect semicircle over the mountain. The sun blinked out, covered by a fast-moving cloud. As the clouds moved, so did the rainbow, disappearing for a moment but then reappearing on the other side of the mountain.

All the while Kate and I sat with a warm sun on our backs, throwing long shadows eastward.

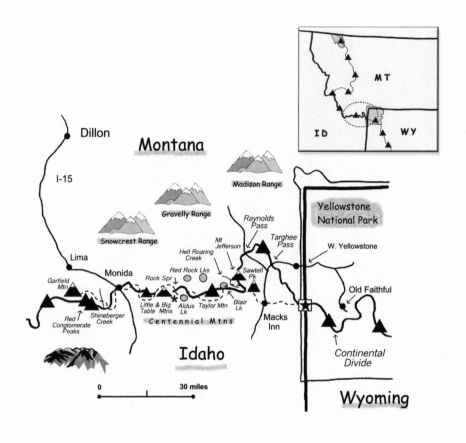

Our hiking route **(Chapter 12)** from Garfield Mountain east to
Yellowstone National Park. Our route is shown as a dashed line.
The inset shows the approximate area included in the larger map.

TWELVE

◤

Choosing a Path

Death is not a failure. Not choosing to take on the challenge of life is.

BERNIE SIEGEL
Love, Medicine and Miracles

K ATE AND I had some trouble finding our way from Garfield
Mountain to Shineberger Creek. The day started with a light rain.
Little tread existed and we fought through tall grass and sticker-
choked brush. Deep scratches soon marked my bare legs. Just below the
Red Conglomerate Peaks, a 30- or 40-mile-per-hour wind hit, a wind that
would stay with us for a couple of hours while we dropped down a long
ridge into Sawmill Creek.

That long ridge pointed us off the Divide toward the high, dry plains
near Monida. An odd bulbous peak called The Thumb joined Garfield
Mountain and the Red Conglomerates to pose a vivid contrast to the
high plains country. Overhead, fast-moving clouds played games with
sun and shadow, carving deep relief into the landscape.

Those views were about all there was to recommend the trip from
Sawmill Creek to Little Beaver Creek. The two-mile walk quickly became
an embarrassment of overgrazing, cow pies, trampled vegetation, and
destroyed riparian zones. Once-delicate creeks now qualified as bombed-
out mud pits.

Sick of cows in the creeks, cows in the forest, cows in the trail, Kate
finally turned verbally abusive, screaming, "Get out of here! Go on, *get*

moving!" Kate swore then and there never to eat a beef burger again. "I will not patronize an industry that destroys the land this way." Though bold and heartfelt, this wasn't a revelation to set the cattle industry quaking. Kate has not eaten beef in years.

Kate's foul mood was not helped by a poorly marked track, nor was mine. Because of the multitude of cow trails, guessing the correct path to follow proved impossible. We finally found one blaze after an exhaustive half-hour hunt, but at Little Beaver Creek our search for the blazed trail over to Shineberger Creek proved fruitless.

For an hour we looked, trying to find a marker that one of our two guidebooks assured us existed. Its description was hazy enough that we finally decided the authors probably had not found the trail either. So why didn't they just say so? Kate, still a little warm under the collar, declared her refusal to use that guidebook for walking through the Centennials. Tired, hungry, and frustrated, we finally chose our own path, setting a compass bearing into the forest and then bushwhacking across several ridges to Shineberger Creek.

A few words about guidebooks: This was Kate's and my first experience hiking with a guidebook—we had two—and we learned a bit during the experience. First, look for a guidebook that tells you what it *doesn't* know. Jim Wolf's CDTS guidebook has shortcomings, sure, but thank God the man tells you when he's reading from the map, or passing along information from another hiker. With *qualified* information you can make reasoned decisions. What hurts is chasing down a path that an author suggests, as we did too many times with our other guidebook, only to find that the landscape was not as it was so assuredly represented.

Second, we learned to be wary of information that was too exact. The guidebook we often questioned sometimes described distances to the hundredth of a mile, as in 16.75 miles. One one-hundredth of a mile equates to 17.6 yards, or roughly 18 steps. Between two guidebooks, maps, trail signs, and our gut feel, we could rarely get mileages to match to two or three miles, much less *hundredths* of a mile.

Taking a guidebook along on your journey is like taking another person. "What does Wolf say?" becomes a frequent question as you stand at an unmarked intersection or at a trail that has just petered out into nothingness. Within this new relationship you soon develop trust or wariness. Trust comes when your guide saves you time, gets the mileages right, suggests an alternative route, or points out something that you might have missed. Trust builds when the author lets you know that a stream crossing and fork in the trail are two miles apart, even though he or she just chose to put them in abutting sentences. True trust has been achieved when you find yourself heading down into a valley that doesn't "feel" right, just because your guide says it's so.

◪

In the world of cancer treatment, good doctors can serve the same function as good guidebooks—making suggestions, presenting options, providing insight based on their knowledge and experience, pointing the way. Good doctors, like good trail guides, tell you what it's like on the trail they have walked, but don't dismiss the possibilities of another path. Good doctors have humility. Good doctors never forget that their advice has a direct influence on your life and hence deserves more than passing consideration. Good doctors tell you what they don't know; they do not pretend to know what is around the next bend if it is a mystery to them. Good doctors are not afraid to speak in shades of gray. Good doctors guide, they do not direct.

Among the most important occurrences in our cancer experience was connecting with Drs. Joanna Cain and Wui-jin Koh. During Kate's time at the University of Washington Medical Center, these two people guided us through the medical morass of cancer treatment. They described the different paths we could travel and the outcomes—both good and bad—that might result from those choices. They made recommendations, but Kate and I never felt we had lost control of our destiny. It is amazing in retrospect to feel such strength of admiration for these people. Even in recalling the agony of Kate's treatments and the burdens she still carries, even as we continue to daily explore alternative pathways, we realize that in our place and time these people did everything they could with the knowledge they had to keep Kate alive. We thank them for those efforts.

Although we often visited with both of our doctors during Kate's regular checkups, as time went by, our interactions with Dr. Cain took center stage. We looked forward in a strange way to our visits—to hearing about her children and to sharing what had happened in our lives since our last visit. Then, roughly a year after Kate's final surgery, Joanna threw us for a loop—she was moving back east. Though our visits to Seattle were becoming less and less frequent, Dr. Cain's move troubled us. Suddenly a ragged tear had formed in our security blanket.

Fittingly, Joanna reintroduced us to Barbara Goff, her oncology partner and a doctor who had shared in Kate's care several times during Kate's hospital stays. Joanna spoke highly of Dr. Goff, and that praise meant a lot to us. We quickly learned that Dr. Goff shared Dr. Cain's ability to connect with Kate. Dr. Goff shared with Drs. Koh and Cain the remarkable talent of being present with Kate, spending her time with Kate without always seeming to be needed somewhere else. We felt, and still feel, blessed to have found a new, trustworthy partner.

There's another way that guidebooks and medical practitioners—whether they come from a Western or alternative medicine approach—are alike: They only work as well as you do. At times on our hike we started down the wrong path only to realize that the error resulted from our poor study of the guidebook, not with some fault of the guide. The medical world is a bit like that.

I believe that doctors respond to informed patients who are courteous, yet demanding. By studying Kate's disease we could participate in its treatment. We could ask and pry and challenge our medical team. We studied Kate's illness the way one might study a map. Where are we pointed? What turns might we make from here? We kept such good records that rather than check Kate's file, our doctors would sometimes ask me for Kate's last red blood cell count or similar data. I believe our doctors reacted to our knowledge. I believe we pushed them to be the best they could for Kate.

Understand that I do not mean to imply that we knew a fraction of what our doctors knew about cancer or the Western approach to treating it, but we knew (and know) two points better than anyone. First, we knew how Kate felt at any given moment, and second, we knew how fervently Kate wanted to get well. Those things sound simple, I know, but they are critical because they form the foundation of Kate's approach to cancer. The most important guide on Kate's return to health is Kate.

No one wanted (or wants) Kate to survive her cancer as much as Kate. She did not abdicate the responsibilities entailed in her hunger for survival. Instead, she fought for her health by learning about her disease, learning to listen to what her body was telling her, changing the makeup of her medical team when she felt it necessary, and controlling her daily interactions and schedule to the point of near total elimination of negative influences. Kate still fights in these ways.

Controlling negative influences proved critical in Kate's climb back to health. We all have realists in our lives, and Kate was no different. She regularly fought off those people who only could talk of false hopes and the imminence of death. Some people facing a life-threatening disease find peace by accepting death. Kate never reached that point.

"Why should I have had to prove to people that I was going to live, when I could barely see that path myself?" Kate asked. "I couldn't be around people who drained my energy. I had to be around energetic, positive people, not downers." And so Kate sought out positive, life-building influences whenever possible, and made substantial efforts to avoid negativity of any kind.

Kate was and is her own best guide, a self-advocate with a purpose. She trusts what she feels and demands the best from those participating in her path to health. She believes that she was and is responsible for her own recovery from cancer and, more broadly, her own well-being.

I recognize that some people might think that all this talk about Kate's role in her recovery and ongoing good health is smoke and mirrors. Perhaps nothing that Kate has done really has mattered. Perhaps she was predestined to survive. Perhaps we have been blessed with six years of life after cancer, but someday the cancer will return.

Perhaps . . . but this is such a defeatist line of reasoning. Kate and I have chosen a less fatalistic path. We believe that much about cancer remains a mystery. We believe that our bodies are magical machines that mankind has only begun to decipher. We believe that inside of that mystery and magic is a place where Kate can exercise control of her health, or at a minimum, maintain an environment conducive to health. It is an approach that leaves the door open to the possibility of life. Perhaps the cancer researchers, the Simontons, stated it best when they wrote:

In the face of uncertainty, there is nothing wrong with hope.

After a night at Shineberger Creek, Kate and I rose at 5 A.M. in hopes of making it out to Monida. The walk would be 19 miles, three miles farther than we'd ever hiked in a single day. We considered breaking the distance into two easy days, but the lure of a hot shower proved too strong.

We ate breakfast by headlamp that morning and then started walking just as a hint of light touched the sky. Kate and I made a beeline for the Divide, climbing straight up the ridge alongside Shineberger Creek. Halfway up, a fiery eastern horizon announced the day's arrival. The faint glow revealed clouds of import moving fast over the Divide. Soon a cold sun arrived to throw flat light across the land. Our shadows fell long off the ridgeline, merging into the darkness that still haunted the ravines below.

Topping out on the barren Divide, the wind hit us like the wash from a jet engine. We both had on, and now kept on, our bright red rain jackets, even though the morning sun was finally taking on the day. The wind raced out of Idaho and into Montana, flattening tufts of bunch grass until they lay parallel to the ground. Ahead, the treeless Divide ebbed and flowed clearly before us. The state boundary fence rode the ridge, looking like a miniature Great Wall of China disappearing into the distance.

Soon we spotted two camouflaged bow hunters struggling up a steep Montana hillside. They paused to sit atop the Divide, clearly bushed. One of them pulled out his binoculars, expecting to look out into the vast dawn loneliness of remote country. The hunter swung his binoculars in a wide arc. Suddenly he went rigid and then he was pointing at the two red-coated aliens moving up the ridgeline. The hunters stood and quickly slid through the fence. By the time we reached their position, the men had slipped off the Divide and disappeared into a stand of trees in Idaho.

Kate and I pushed on through the morning, for a time following OHV tracks and at other times walking without the benefit of any tread. Sometimes the Divide plummeted so steeply that as we hiked down off the ridgetop our thigh muscles burned. "Down," we had long ago learned, is never without recourse in CDT walking. Soon enough we would be scaling another steep rise. For hours we rolled up and down. The Divide was a *Stegosaurus* and we were hiking along its spine.

The wind continued to pound the ridge, seemingly in a grand rush to get from the Pacific to the Atlantic. We hid in a depression on the Montana side of the Divide for our first lunch at 10:30. Soon the wind ratcheted up another notch. We leaned hard over Idaho to keep from blowing into the fence. Once Kate yelled and I looked back to see her pinned on the barbwire. I ran back and extracted her. Both of us were happy to find she had only cut her pants, not her legs. Climbing steeply up the next hill, the gale rocked Kate so hard that I walked beside her to act as a windbreak. Kate put her arm through mine and we climbed to the next rise like newlyweds walking up the wedding aisle.

We walked ever east into the sun until finally turning north into Horse Creek and thus, at long last, putting the wind at our back. As we dropped to the creek the wind fell away, the trail turned to a flat, soft road, and the temperature rose to a healthy level. We ate a second lunch and then pounded out the now easy miles.

Because of the improved conditions, we quickly realized that this was *not* to be an epic day, that indeed we would make Monida by day's end. Soon we spotted our first real CDT reassurance sign in days—if not weeks—and shouted in joy. We grew giddy. Once, getting far ahead, I mooned Kate across the miles of sagebrush. I could see her chuckling in the distance. A few miles on we began to see semi trucks, and then later cars on I-15. Behind us an apocalyptic storm brewed over the Lima Peaks. Gigantic purple clouds, trailing long veils to the ground, seemed to signal the end of the world. Elsewhere shafts of sunlight highlighted empty hills and prairie.

After crossing the I-15 fences, we placed a marker where we hit the frontage road—our starting place after a few days of rest—then turned north to Monida. Monida, a dusty near–ghost town of four or five houses and a few deserted buildings, sits astride the Divide and the Montana-Idaho border. In the second half of the 18th century, Monida was born as a stagecoach stop between Salt Lake City and the booming Montana goldmines. The town's name, which comes from a combination of the words "Montana" and "Idaho," came later with the laying of the Utah and Northern Railroad tracks. For a time early in this century tourists came north to Monida by train, then boarded red stagecoaches for the overland trip to Yellowstone National Park.

One of Monida's remaining houses belonged to Clay Roselle, the owner of Monida's only active business, a junkyard. My folks had shuttled our car to Clay's place weeks earlier. Kate and I had also been to Clay's house once before, on a scouting journey, but had yet to meet him.

The house's environs had undergone a considerable transformation since that first visit of ours. No more dented school buses or rusted car bodies surrounded the house—in fact, no junk was visible at all. Everything had been bladed clean to soil as if a small nuclear attack had been waged on Montana's southern border.

Clay greeted us when we came to collect our car. A bearded man, he was wearing an oily ball cap and dirty overalls. Clay explained that he had moved all the car bodies and oil drums and old parts from his yard up onto the hill with the rest of the junkyard.

Months earlier, in Lima, a local had told us that Clay has all the junk inventoried in his brain. "He's amazing. You can go up to Clay's junkyard there and find just about anything. Ask him, he'll find it tucked away under the seat of some broken-down bus out back. 'Round here, we call it 'Clay-Mart.'"

Kate and I bid Clay thanks, then collected our car in the Clay-Mart parking lot and headed north. We took a big break then—four days—traveling to Elk Horn Hot Springs and Missoula before returning to the trail at Monida. In Missoula, Patricia, our new friend from the Pintlers, and her husband, Gary, welcomed us to their home on the side of Mount Jumbo. They treated us like royalty with morning coffee, special desserts, and even a party given in our honor. Patricia fed our minds, too, with well-thought-out theories on the CDT, Lewis and Clark, and the opening of the West.

While at Patricia and Gary's, Kate and I spent a bit of time reviewing the toll that 725 miles of hiking had taken on our gear: two pairs of delaminated boots, two leaking tents, a broken fly rod, a lost knife. . . .

The list of gear casualties went on to more than a dozen items, but in truth the losses brought us little sorrow. Gear is gear, nothing more. Gear is a tool to aid in an experience. Unfortunately, in these marketeer-driven days, people too often confuse gear *for* the experience. We've left lots of gear behind and we look forward to having more, but the things we truly value now more than ever carry no price tag.

◪

Over the years since Kate's last surgery, her periodic checkups have changed from once a month to every two, three, and then six months. Over time the butterfly period—that time when our stomachs quake at just the thought of returning to Seattle and what we might learn there— has decreased again and again until now our stomachs only go raw the day before Kate's appointment.

During some of Kate's more recent checkups, I've at times become overwhelmed with the thought that we simply did not belong at the Cancer Center anymore. Our lives were moving on. Sometimes our doctors have looked almost relieved to see us, as if maybe we were a break in the midst of a day where so many other patient problems loomed. Sometimes I find that I have forgotten the terminology of cancer. And we no longer recognize many of the people in the Women's Clinic or Cancer Center. At one recent checkup, now several years since Joanna Cain's departure from UWMC, a new resident came in to interview us before Dr. Goff arrived. When we spoke of a recent conversation with Dr. Cain, the unknowing resident asked, "And so what did *he* have to say?"

Almost five years after Kate's final surgery, it was even suggested that if we wanted we could change the time between Kate's regular checkups from six months to one year. Yes, our lives were moving on, yet Kate and

I had the same reaction to that suggestion: "No!" Neither of us was or is ready to lose contact with the folks who have directed Kate's medical path to health. Most important, if another problem ever—God forbid—occurs, we see great value in receiving the earliest possible warning.

◪

Thirty pronghorns watched as Kate and I started back onto the trail at Monida after our four days of rest. We hiked along the interstate, then turned up Long Creek and climbed through tinder-dry grasses. Six miles on we found a surging spring and dropped our packs. It was a short but productive day, putting us back on the trail for the last segment of our hike across Montana and the last days of summer. Simply getting re-started on a day like that was the goal, not making miles.

The next couple of days we pushed into the Centennial Mountains. The Centennials are a 50-mile-long escarpment that rises gently—like a water ski jump—out of Idaho's Snake River Plains. For miles the mountains climb, slowly but to staggering heights, until at their northerly edge the Centennials abruptly crash down to Montana's Red Rock Lakes thousands of feet below. On the west end of the Centennials we walked only on the gentle upslope, at first through golden grasses, then later through pine forests. By now most of the flowers had faded and drooped. Pockets of yellowing aspens showed. Fall may have been officially a week away, but on the Divide it had started rounding into shape.

We crossed the edge of Little Table Mountain without the aid of a trail, dropping through deep buckbrush and downed timber. At the Pete Creek Divide, we finally came back onto a footpath and even saw some CDT reassurance symbols. For a brief spurt the symbols came every third tree, as if a trail crew had wanted to use up their allotment of signs and close out the workday as rapidly as possible. Kate and I felt excited to be on a dedicated hiking trail, the first real hiking trail we'd been on since near Deadman Lake roughly 50 miles earlier.

Our excitement didn't last long, however. The trail quickly disappeared again into the nothingness of mixed forest and meadow. We looked hard numerous times before finding some old tree blazes along the southern edge of Big Table Mountain. Our long searches proved futile, however, because downed timber littered the scant sections of trail that we did find. Kate and I pinballed our way along, never quite sure if we were headed in the right direction, sometimes searching for and magically finding blazes, sometimes giving up on the blazes and choosing to follow the compass. Eventually we found our way into a sagebrush meadow where a strong track finally returned.

Shortly after entering the meadow, we came to East Camas Creek. We dropped the packs and paused for a moment's rest. Suddenly Kate grew excited and, pointing, she exclaimed, "Look! The Tetons!" Far in the distance stood the hazy, familiar outlines of those marvelous mountains.

Kate and I had once listened to an arrogant man speak about an overland bicycle tour. The man started by describing his earlier kayaking escapades, then said, "Once I became famous in kayaking circles, I decided I wanted to become famous in bicycling circles." People in the crowd looked at each other as if to say, "Who does this guy think he is, anyway?"

Kate and I have joked about that man's comment many times since then. Here now, newly rejuvenated by the view of the Tetons, Kate spoke boastfully—facetiously—in a way she shares only with me.

"I walked here from Canada, you know," she beamed. "Almost 800 miles." I gave her an astonished look. "No, really. I did. It's true. And now I can see the Tetons!" All this was spoken with a highly self-satisfied smile.

"Wow, so tell me," I asked mockingly, "how does it feel to be famous in hiking circles?"

We camped a night at Rock Spring, which trickled timidly from a pipe, and then another night at Aldus Lake, where a lone elk bugled from dusk until dawn. On the trail, grasshoppers by the thousands scattered from our path, so incredibly awkward in their efforts at flight. Sometimes the hoppers landed on our legs; always their odd chatter surrounded us.

Once we came upon a substantial set of bear tracks. Soon we crossed an equally substantial pile of bear scat, fresh bear scat. Then, shortly before Ching Creek, Kate stopped suddenly and took two hurried steps back. As I started to ask if she'd seen a bear, the woods resounded with the crash of a large, running animal. Wide-eyed, Kate said yes, and that it had been an especially large black bear and that as it ran away she'd had an especially good look at its large rump. We yelled and moved ahead, but saw no sign of the bear again.

Not far beyond Aldus Lake, roughly halfway across the Centennials, we walked into the vast grasslands of the Agricultural Service's Sheep Research Station. The open views revealed Baldy and Slide Mountains, and for the first time hints of the Centennials' sheer escarpment face.

We had already hiked a dozen miles that day but chose, stupidly, to start up 9,855-foot Taylor Mountain. Hours later, on top the Divide and feeling worn, we peered over the escarpment's edge to see rocky crags falling into nothingness. Red Rock Lakes sat silently before us, 3,000 feet below and yet barely a horizontal mile away. Farther north, the Snowcrest and Gravelly Ranges showed. To the east, more mountains—Nemesis and Jefferson and Sawtell—glowed pink in the late sun. But I think my favorite view was across Island Park Reservoir, so vast and flat, and beyond that to the Tetons. Clouds blanketed the entire scene in dark shadows, yet the top half of the Tetons glowed from a hidden sun.

All this beauty brought Kate and me less jubilation than usual. Both of us had agonized through the long climb up Taylor Mountain. Kate's feet and hips ached. The fact that she admitted so was a sure sign that things were very bad. For Kate, every step up the mountain became an act of courage—one foot in front of the other; step-by-step to the top. I drew strength from Kate. I felt sore myself, largely because of the eight pounds of water we'd thrown on my back at our morning break. It was the last accessible water we expected to see for 15 or 20 miles.

Fully spent, we stopped that night high on a bare ridge above Keg Spring Road. It was not the best camp we had ever selected. A cold south wind assaulted our position. Rocks and bunchgrass lumped the ground under the tent. But we felt too tired to proceed. We had chosen to put in over nine hours of walking for the third consecutive day. It was simply too much for us. After three months on the trail, we should have been smarter.

At midmorning the next day, Kate and I stopped at Blair Lake to undertake a serious "summit." For a week we had been discussing whether we should follow the CDT proper over Raynolds and Targhee Passes or instead take the shorter route favored by Wolf. Wolf's route, taken by all the CDT hikers we had met, headed directly from near Blair Lake to Mack's Inn, Idaho. Wolf's route knocked 25 or 30 miles off the hike by shortcutting the Divide's last northward bump into Montana. By heading for Mack's Inn—and previously taking the Anaconda Cutoff— our Montana CDT walk would total roughly 810 miles, rather than the official trail length of around 900 miles.

For an hour Kate and I mulled over the topo maps. Kate favored the shorter Mack's Inn route; I favored the Targhee Pass route. Still, there was the threat of September snow, plus a 10,000-foot Divide crossing on the longer route. Also, our map showed a faint trail labeled "CONST" on the Targhee Pass route. Did the Forest Service simply misspell "CDNST" for "Continental Divide National Scenic Trail," we wondered, or were they trying to indicate "trail under construction?"

In the end we chose to forgo the unknown. Going with Wolf assured us of finishing the journey on a high note. Also, the lure of following in the footsteps of the other CDT hikers we had met intrigued us. And though it wasn't stated out loud, it didn't escape me that we would finish the journey in the same way we started it, under Kate's edict, "Well, we haven't done anything stupid yet. Let's not start now."

◪

"In the face of uncertainty, there is nothing wrong with hope."

Those are powerful words. Hope is critical in healing from cancer. Focusing on the positive, on that which is hopeful, and declaring control of her own life have provided Kate a handhold to lift herself back to health.

Recently, Kate wrote an ailing friend a note that reflects this philosophy:

> *I was freaked out about bodily stuff, too—hair falling out, bloated belly, swelled legs, and not being able to eat for two months. If I*

thought about it I cried. A little denial and ignoring those problems helped me spend time thinking about happier things.

I can understand why you are not feeling very happy. I know it feels like there is no clear solution and that feels disempowering. I think it's good to cry it out until you're sick of crying. Then look for and find and focus on the hopeful part.

After about a month of depression I suddenly was SICK and TIRED of being everyone's Ping-Pong ball and having them tell me what was going to happen. I thought, "Dammit, I'm in control of this. I don't have to listen to these people tell me I'm going to die. I can control every decision and every input and I can get better." That was the first time I actually envisioned the path where I would get well and felt I had a decent chance of getting there.

◪

The decision to head for Mack's Inn gave our legs new life. Off we went on a newly marked trail, down into a valley where Wolf's route broke with the CDT. Soon we started up vibrant Hell Roaring Creek and the trail petered out. Still we marched ahead confidently as Wolf hit every description. As she had done in the past, Kate commended Wolf on his "nerdlike enthusiasm." I suggested she be slow to hand out that label, given that she had just walked for two hours with one pant leg tucked in her sock.

Higher and higher we climbed until Hell Roaring Creek diminished to a trickle. Soon we stood beside the creek's first timorous drips. Certainly this must be the highest point on the most distant tributary of the Missouri. We stopped to consider the grand journey those droplets would take to the Gulf of Mexico, a journey that knew not of defeat, but instead looked ahead with hope and a great belief in possibilities.

Kate and I touched those first drops, hugged, then climbed easily onto the Divide. Not far along, we set up camp on a ridge overlooking the Yellowstone Plateau. A cold wind howled up from the valley. Heavy storm clouds hung overhead. The clouds grew pink, then purple, then gunmetal blue as the sun dropped lower and lower. Above us on Sawtell

Peak's skyline stood the glowing white sphere of an FAA control center. At dusk, car lights heading down the darkened face of the mountain from the obelisk gave our camp a decidedly outer space feel.

We ate late, after dark. Back in Glacier in June, we'd read by natural light until 10:30 every night. Here on the edge of the Centennials, just days before the fall equinox, darkness came early. By 8 we needed a headlamp to close down camp for the night.

We shivered into the tent. It was our last night camping on the CDT and we talked like two kids at a slumber party. I told Kate I barely remembered what I had been doing at work just three and half short months earlier. Kate said she remembered, but that she never thought of it much. We talked about missing our cat. We talked about the landscape we had just passed through, and how Montana suited us better than any place we had ever lived or visited. We talked about what we would do in the months ahead, what we would do when the walk and the summer ended.

Transitions are important times. Whenever an important segment of our lives nears completion, Kate and I talk about the afterward. We lay out the possibilities for the future, postulate silly ideas, walk mentally down a hundred paths, dream. For a short time cancer robbed us of our ability to look to the future. Many nights in the Montana backcountry, Kate and I thanked God for the good health to walk 800 miles, and for giving us back the capacity to dream.

We woke that last morning on the Divide to a beautiful, uniquely Rocky Mountain sight: a golden sunrise in the midst of a snowstorm. Frozen condensation made the tent fly brittle. Winter clouds—cold clouds— scraped the top of Sawtell Peak, but below them a giant, chilly sun sent daggers of light into the world. Looking out from the tent, I was reminded of the old Montana saying "If you don't like the weather, just wait five minutes."

I didn't wait. I stepped into the falling snow, caught some of it on my outstretched tongue, and then in the words of a friend I shouted to the mountains, "It's gonna be a golden day!" Indeed, we were only halfway down Sawtell Peak when the warming sun claimed the day as its own. Soon we doffed our jackets and gloves.

The snow seemed a fitting way to close down our hike across Montana. There were two more days until the first day of fall, the day we would walk to the border of Yellowstone Park and the hike's end. As we walked and talked, Kate and I marveled at the weather we had experienced over the summer. Racking our brains, we could only come up with eight rain days on the trail, and four of those occurred during the tough first two weeks in Glacier.

Down onto the pavement, near Mack's Inn, Kate and I pushed through a thousand sheep being driven to winter pasture. Horsemen nodded at us while purposeful dogs nipped the mob into line. When the road narrowed the mob squeezed in, and we became boulders in a stream of wet, dank wool. Kate and I laughed as we waded upstream toward the end of the hike, slowed but still moving ahead.

◤

Living beyond cancer—like living with cancer—is a challenge. Living beyond cancer entails choice. Kate realized early on that she could either choose to focus forever on the valley behind her, or instead turn to embrace the mountains ahead.

Fear, anger, and a sense of loss have sometimes permeated our beings. At times in the years since Kate's last treatment our fear has been palpable, especially when hearing stories about people whose cancer—including cervical adenocarcinoma—has returned 5, 10, even 15 years after successful treatment. Fear comes, too, as we agonize through the pain of others' cancer experiences, and sometimes through their deaths.

For a time we held deep anger at the lax approach we felt our early doctors took toward Kate's "lymphocyst" which, sadly, turned out to be recurrent cancer. Tied up in that resentment was anger *at ourselves* for not demanding to see our Portland oncologist sooner. Why did other doctors tell us they would have done things differently? Why didn't we understand how serious all this was? Why did we want to deny? Would Kate be suffering the agonies of poor digestive function and lymphedema if we had simply acted faster? And what if we had forgone the medical route altogether and instead put our faith in the body's power to heal itself?

"For a long time," Kate told me, "I was angry at our doctor for mistaking my tumor for a lymphocyst. Changing doctors dealt with that mistake in a hurry. Now I realize that he was doing his best, had good intentions, and is a fragile human just like the rest of us. I wouldn't go to him again as a doctor because I think his approach was too cavalier, but I forgive him for the mistake."

Fear, anger, and a sense of loss could control Kate today, but only if she chose to allow them to. I don't pretend to say that these emotions were and are not real, or appropriate, or even necessary. We still cry sometimes about today's agonies and yesterday's memories. But shortly after the cancer treatments ended, the question became this: Just how long will we allow these emotions to control us?

In *Love, Medicine and Miracles*, Bernie Siegel writes:

> *We have an infinite number of choices ahead,*
> *but a finite number of endings.*

Among those infinite choices is one that for Kate and me can be boiled down to this: I accept what has happened to me and I mourn those things which cancer has taken from me, but today I will begin my journey forward, today I will release my anger and fear and choose to live.

Making that choice set the tone for how we live today. Here's a perfect example: People have said to Kate, "Wow, you've been in remission for five years. That's great, congratulations!"

We—at least I—will quietly inform these people that no, in fact Kate's cancer is not in "remission." Kate's cancer is *gone*. For people that have no measurable tumor, like Kate, *remission* is a coldly defeatist word that puts a damper on any progress. Remission puts one in an eternal holding pattern, since the inference is clearly that the cancer is simply waiting to come back. If—God forbid—Kate's cancer ever returns, for Kate and me it will be new cancer. Instead of fear and waiting, Kate early on chose a path of joy and progress.

Pogo, the cartoon character, strikes this same chord with a slightly different mallet, saying:

> *We are confronted with insurmountable opportunities.*

How then would we choose to see life, we asked ourselves, as a trail ending abruptly at a cliff or as one that marches on toward limitless horizons? The choice, Kate and I realized, sat with us. And in the end, importantly, it was a choice that did not require cancer as a balance point.

◪

Mack's Inn, Idaho, a tiny settlement on the banks of the Henry's Fork of the Snake River, is for many the figurative end to the Montana section of their CDT hike. During the months we planned for the hike, however, Kate and I had always focused on finishing at the boundary of Yellowstone National Park. Though we had opted to follow Wolf's path to Mack's Inn instead of following the CDT past Raynolds and Targhee Passes, we still wanted to finish at Yellowstone.

We broke that final 17 miles—from Mack's Inn to the Yellowstone boundary—into two segments, both of which traveled mostly along gravel roads. Most of the forest we passed through was sparse. Some of it had been logged; much had been scorched by the Yellowstone fires of 1988.

Even in this relative austerity, however, I felt a simultaneous sense of beauty and loss. I wanted to remember everything those final two days, to hold on to the hike in a way that I would never lose it. I recall trying to stuff it all into my mind, hoping to remember forever the clouds hanging quietly over Island Park, the light dusting of snow on the Henrys Mountains, the golden eagle soaring along the ridgeline above us, the way the grass waved in the wind, the reflection of the sun off the creek, the burst of fall colors.

Kate and I played a game as we walked, asking each other, "What was the hardest day of the hike? The easiest? The coldest? The hottest? What was the best meal? The scariest moment? The most welcome beer?"

I asked Kate if she remembered our friend Linda's card, from way back at the start of the hike, a card that showed a little boy sitting in front of his house, fishing pole in hand, pulling fish after fish from a curbside puddle. "Remember," I said, "inside, the card read, 'All great things begin with a dream.'"

Kate looked at me with a smile and replied, "Yep, and with a little stubbornness, too."

*   *   *

It struck me on our final day, as we walked three miles in to touch the Yellowstone border, that finishing an 810-mile walk did not mean we could stop worrying about cancer. It did not mean that we could skip our next doctor's appointment (My God, was it only three weeks away?!). Just the previous week, Kate had suffered from excruciating bowel pain that left her crying and writhing on the ground and left me wondering how we could possibly transport her out from deep in the Centennials.

No, finishing the hike did not mean we could forget about cancer. Finishing the walk did not mean we could stop our diligent efforts at eating a healthy diet and at keeping Kate's immune system strong. We had not "conquered" cancer but—perhaps more importantly—maybe finishing the hike proved that neither had cancer conquered us. Maybe, just maybe, I thought, what finishing our walk across Montana did was show us that we still had choices, and that the strength of the spirit is more important than the strength of a physical affliction.

We crossed a small ravine, then came to the base of a hill. A large, newly posted reassurance symbol showed that our trail was merging back into the Continental Divide Trail proper. We followed the CDT up the hill, then came to a wide swath cut through the trees. On the far side of that boundary clear-cut, Yellowstone's untouched forests waited.

Kate and I hooted and slapped hands as we made our way across the clear-cut. At the forest's edge we found a sign that said U.S. National Park Service Boundary. Putting our arms around each other, we counted to three, then took one giant shared step into Yellowstone.

EPILOGUE

◤

But who expected bumblebees could fly? Oh go ahead and fly . . .

CHRISTINE LAVIN
"Miracle of Bumblebee Flight"

D URING THE EARLY STAGES of preparing this book, Kate went through her five-year posttreatment checkup at the University of Washington Medical Center. Kate's medical team and I had a small surprise celebration planned for after the exam.

Thankfully, the checkup went perfectly. When Kate's oncologist, Barbara Goff, finished the exam, she said, "You just go ahead and get dressed because I have to step out to . . . ah . . . ah . . . do *something* in the hall." Kate threw me a quizzical look as if to say, "She sure is acting oddly today."

Moments later Dr. Goff returned with several of the nurses—Jana, Katy, Holly, and Heidi—who had been so important in Kate's hospital care. Dr. Koh arrived shortly. Dr. Goff, smiling, presented Kate with a book about climbing Everest, a book that many of Kate's caregivers, including Dr. Cain, had signed. Kate seemed stunned. She was speechless, her eyes wide and wet with tears.

Jana brought out some sparkling apple cider and soon everyone held a glass aloft. Dr. Goff proposed a toast, one whose sentiments included congratulating Kate on five years of being cancer-free and congratulating her on surviving not only cancer, but recurrent cancer. Kate was an

263

inspiration, Dr. Goff said, one that helped keep all of them—doctors and nurses—fighting to assist others in their struggles with cancer. Dr. Goff's voice choked a bit as she spoke, and I could not help but see how important that moment was for everyone, not just Kate and me.

◢

Cancer demands absolute humility. Cancer cannot be ignored, or simply willed away. Its power and possibility live in every moment of the day—for Kate, for me, for you. During one of the darkest moments of our struggle with cancer, in a place where death seemed closer than life and Kate's body seemed to be escaping her, Kate told me, "Love is the only real thing, everything else doesn't really matter."

As the days of the horror cancer brought us grow more distant, we feel a duty to both the daunting humility caused by cancer and to the love of friends and family that is so instrumental in overcoming it. We've chosen to express that duty in ways that we hope can help others. This book is one way. Kate's involvement with the American Cancer Society is another.

Living beyond cancer involves joy and agony. Kate and I laugh with friends and carry on with those things that are dear to us. Sometimes our lives seem almost back to normal. This, of course, is my perception. Kate fights with her bowels and bladder and lymphedema and never has the luxury of seeing things as truly "normal" again. But for me sometimes days go by where thoughts of cancer barely cross my mind. Still, the cancer is always there—growing hazy like a grizzly's outline in the mist, perhaps, yet never disappearing—and sometimes something will happen which pointedly reminds me of cancer's presence. Near the end of our hike such a moment occurred.

We were partway through the Centennials, walking late in the day. Both of us felt leg-weary from the day's miles and from walking an endless sidehill with no trail. As the sun dropped another notch, Kate stopped, unknown to me. I walked ahead, pushing hard, lost in my own thoughts.

Past a couple of corners I thought to look back. Kate was nowhere in sight. I paused for a time, then finally took off my pack and sat. I felt tired and sore and had little desire to backtrack to find her. As the wait grew longer and longer, thoughts of sprained ankles and mountain lions crept into my mind. Finally the time came—we had rarely been separated on the trail this long—and I started back.

After a few steps, I drew up, feeling an abrupt pang in my stomach. What if she's not coming? I thought. What if the cancer has taken her and all I will ever do again is look down an empty trail into a cold wind? The trail stayed silent and my eyes welled with tears. Thank God for the time we have shared together was all I could think in answer. Thank God for giving us twin spirits that desire to live substantially.

I blinked away the tears and then suddenly there rounding the corner came Kate, marching steadily up the trail, implacable as ever, a smile on her face.

ACKNOWLEDGMENTS

◪

MANY, MANY people had a hand in bringing this book into being. Attempting to thank everyone who made some impact on the book is an impossible task. I will almost surely forget someone in the words that follow, and for that I am truly sorry. Friends and family provided encouragement countless times during the preparation of this book. Their love and good thoughts mattered, providing me a solid foundation for continued effort and work. I humbly thank each of them for their support.

I want to thank Linda Ashkenas, who read the book's earliest version. Much of the book's flow and many of its central themes are rooted in comments that originally came from Linda. In many spots in the text, I can see where Linda's words somehow magically became my words. Her suggestions run through the book like a stream runs through a valley—right at its heart and center. Linda helped me through some tearful times as I wrote, much as she did during the depth of Kate's and my cancer experience. Linda, I thank you for your wisdom, talent, time, and friendship.

Friends Kathy Brewer and Chris Slater provided valuable input after the book's second rendering. They tackled a work still in tremendous need of refinement. Thanks to Kathy for many thoughtful suggestions and conversations on content and direction. Thanks to Chris for careful editing and commentary. The book moved to a higher plane because of Kathy and Chris's adept skills, prolific reading habits, and flair for the written word.

Thanks to the many other friends who gave freely of their time to read later editions of the book and provide valuable feedback: Frank Bretl and

Anne Reiling, Jeff Igelman and Theresa Gibney, Colleen Llewellyn, Annette Simonson, Rachel Potter, Polly Burke, and Jim and Marie Neale, who sent good thoughts from Australia. Thanks to friend and photographer Eric Hansen for his encouragement. Thanks to friend Betsy Buffington for providing her unique perspectives on health and wilderness. Thanks to friend Chris Beatty at Ecopress for his wise insight into the endless array of questions I asked about the publishing business, and to both he and Lori Tully for valuable thoughts on the text.

Many people gave freely of their technical expertise. Thanks to Norm Bishop for information on wolves in Yellowstone and Idaho; Dr. Joanna Cain for review of the medically intensive sections of the book; Arnold Dood and Helga Pac of Montana Fish, Wildlife and Parks and Mark Haroldson of the Interagency Grizzly Bear Study Team, for information on the status of grizzly bears in Montana; Janelle Smith at the National Interagency Fire Center in Boise for her help in sorting out the facts and figures of the 1998 fire season in the Northern Rockies; Kim Davitt at American Wildlands for information on the Thunderbolt Blowdown; Deirdre Shaw at Glacier National Park's Museum and Archives for help with the history of Glacier names; Frank Gosar at KLCC in Eugene, Oregon, for help tracking down some of the songs quoted in the book, songs that Kate and I listened to on countless trips to the hospital in Seattle; and postmaster Lisa Martini for forwarding on a copy of the CDT logbook from Leadore, Idaho.

Thanks to Paula and Bruce Ward at the Continental Divide Trail Alliance for their support of this project, for use of a CDTA map, and especially for their passion for completing and protecting the CDT.

Kate and I would like to thank our family members for their feedback and input into the book. As importantly, we thank them for understanding that by allowing a small piece of *their* lives to be revealed in this story, they are helping us in our attempt to help others.

Thanks to three readers—Gloria Flora, Walkin' Jim Stoltz, and Bill Cunningham—for their willingness to spend their valuable time reviewing a story that had no publisher when they agreed to read it and that came from an author they barely knew. The gratitude Kate and I feel for their help is matched only by our admiration for the incredible efforts each of them has made to protect our remaining wildlands. Similarly, thanks to Ross Rogers, another champion of the wilderness, a fishing mate and, as it turns out, one heck of an editor.

I would like to thank the good people at the American Cancer Society for believing that our story held merit for helping those dealing with cancer. Thanks to Emily Pualwan for her willingness to listen to an unknown story from an unknown author. Thanks to Kathy Bruss for skillfully overseeing the editorial production of the book and especially for her boundless patience in dealing with my endless questions. Thanks to Chuck Westbrook for his careful review and wise suggestions. Thanks to Candace Magee for her enthusiasm and talents in creating the book's final appearance and to Dana Wagner for work on the book's photographs and maps. Thanks to medical editors Terri Ades and Rick Alteri for their valuable input, and to Tom Gryczan for proofreading.

And perhaps my greatest thanks go to Amy Sproull Brittain, my editor from ACS. Amy polished the rough stone of my writing to as fine a luster as possible. She worked and sweated and prodded and pampered (sorry, Amy, I know there are no commas here, but at least the verbs are active!) and in short did everything possible to make our story come alive on the page. Any shortcomings that remain are mine. Amy's skills helped mold the book far beyond the editing process, beyond even suggestions about methods of storytelling and structure, and indeed extended right into helping me reveal the book's soul. Amy, Kate and I appreciate your talents and, more importantly, appreciate you as a new friend.

And finally to Kate. In allowing your story to be shared with others, you continue to show a level of courage and selflessness that is nearly unfathomable to the rest of us. My heart swells with pride and joy at the privilege of being your partner. You are my inspiration.

SUGGESTED READING

Ambrose, Stephen E. *Undaunted Courage: Meriwether Lewis, Thomas Jefferson, and the Opening of the American West.* New York: Touchstone Books, 1997.

Asher, Michael. *Impossible Journey: Two Against the Sahara.* New York: Penguin Books, 1991.

Berger, Karen and Daniel R. Smith. *Where the Waters Divide: A Walk Along America's Continental Divide.* Nevada City, CA: Harmony Books, 1993.

Brooks, Tad and Sherry Jones. *The Hiker's Guide to Montana's Continental Divide Trail.* Helena, MT: Falcon Press, 1990.

Cahill, Tim. *Pecked to Death by Ducks.* New York: Vintage Books, 1994.

Crichton, Michael. *Travels.* New York: Ballantine Books, 1993.

Cunningham, Bill. *Montana's Continental Divide (Montana Geographic Series* volume number 12). Helena, MT: Montana Magazine, 1986.

Davidson, Robyn. *Tracks.* New York: Pantheon Books, 1980.

Doig, Ivan. *Dancing at the Rascal Fair.* New York: Scribner, 1996.

Doig, Ivan. *English Creek.* New York: Penguin Books, 1985.

Dufresne, Frank. *No Room for Bears.* Anchorage, AK: Alaska Northwest Books, 1991.

Evans, Laura. *The Climb of My Life: A Miraculous Journey from the Edge of Death to the Victory of a Lifetime.* San Francisco: Harper San Francisco, 1996.

Glover, James M. *A Wilderness Original: The Life of Bob Marshall.* Seattle, WA: The Mountaineers, 1986.

Howard, Lynna and Leland, Contintental Divide Trail Alliance. *Montana and Idaho's Continental Divide Trail: The Official Guide (The Continental Divide Trail Series).* Englewood, CO: Westcliffe, 2000.

Jardine, Ray. *The Pacific Crest Trail Hiker's Handbook.* LaPine, OR: AdventureLore Press, 1996.

Lopez, Barry. *Of Wolves and Men.* New York: Charles Scribner's Sons, 1978.

Owens, Mark and Delia. *Cry of the Kalahari.* Boston: Houghton Mifflin Company, 1984.

Peacock, Doug. *Grizzly Years: In Search of the American Wilderness.* New York: Zebra Books, 1992.

Rawlings, Marjorie Kinnan. *The Yearling.* New York: Aladdin, 1998.

Siegel, Bernie. *Love, Medicine and Miracles: Lessons Learned About Self-Healing from a Surgeon's Experience with Exceptional Patients.* New York: Harper Perennial, 1986.

Simonton, O. Carl, Stephanie Matthews-Simonton, and James L. Creighton. *Getting Well Again.* New York: Bantam Books, 1992.

Whyte, David. *The Heart Aroused: Poetry and the Preservation of the Soul in Corporate America.* New York: Currency/Doubleday, 1996.

Williams, Terry Tempest. *Refuge: An Unnatural History of Family and Place.* New York: Vintage Books, 1991.

Wolf, James R. *Guide to the Continental Divide Trail Volume I: Northern Montana.* Baltimore: Continental Divide Trail Society, 1992.

Wolf, James R. *Guide to the Continental Divide Trail Volume II: Southern Montana and Idaho.* Baltimore: Continental Divide Trail Society, 1979.

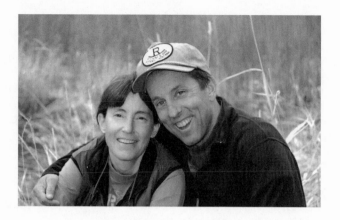

ABOUT THE AUTHOR

Scott Bischke is a writer, environmental engineer, fly fisherman, photographer, and dreamer. He and his wife Katie have traveled across the globe to places like New Zealand, British Columbia, Alaska, Baja, Costa Rica, and Belize in search of the peace, solitude, and tranquility of the natural world.

Since hiking across Montana, Scott and Katie have also backpacked the length of the Continental Divide across Wyoming and Colorado. They plan to cross New Mexico next and thus finish hiking the Continental Divide Trail from Canada to Mexico.

Crossing Divides is Scott's second book. The first, *Two Wheels Around New Zealand: A Bicycle Journey on Friendly Roads*, is a light-hearted travelogue about the year he and Katie spent traveling Down Under.

Scott and Katie are currently self-employed. They consult in the engineering and computer science worlds, and Scott is involved in numerous writing projects.

The couple actively participates in volunteer efforts for the Montana Wilderness Association, the Continental Divide Trail Alliance, and the American Cancer Society, as well as other worthwhile organizations.

Scott and Katie live—most joyously—in Bozeman, Montana.